The Truths and Myths of Weight Loss

The Scientific Evidence

by

Henry W. Snead, M.D.

authorHOUSE®

AuthorHouse™
1663 Liberty Drive, Suite 200
Bloomington, IN 47403
www.authorhouse.com
Phone: 1-800-839-8640

© 2007 Henry W. Snead, M.D.. All rights reserved.

No part of this book may be reproduced, stored in a retrieval system, or transmitted by any means without the written permission of the author.

First published by AuthorHouse 6/11/2007

ISBN: 978-1-4343-1598-4 (sc)

Printed in the United States of America
Bloomington, Indiana

This book is printed on acid-free paper.

CHAPTER OUTLINE

INTRODUCTION:

PROLOGUE:

CHAPTER 1: PSYCHOLOGICAL PASSIONS

Many obese individuals have a history of childhood abuse (sexual, mental or physical) that has led to learned helplessness. This in turn leads to high levels of mood disorders (depression and anxiety) seen in the obese which in turn leads to negative assumptions about the self with a sense of vulnerability. "Disinhibited" eating is the grief reaction for a sense of loss of control.

CHAPTER 2: METABOLIC MYSTERIES

There are metabolic adaptations that occur to prevent weight loss, these adaptations are reviewed in the context of total energy expenditure, centering around the changes in resting metabolic rate, and how these changes which resist weight loss persist for years afterwards, meaning that commitment doesn't stop after the new weight is obtained.

CHAPTER 3: EXERCISE ESCAPADES

Here the failure of increasing energy expenditure with exercise to produce accelerated weight loss is shown to be countered by compensatory decreases in the resting metabolic rate. An interesting graphic presentation with the Boston Police Force is given. This is a major point! Adding exercise to diet doesn't increase weight loss significantly.

CHAPTER 4: REGAIN RAMPAGE

The decreased metabolic rate that accompanies weight loss persists for many years afterwards resulting in the need to eat less or exercise more than those at the same weight who have not lost. Simply put, one maintains weight loss through exercise or you are doomed to regain.

CHAPTER 5: HOMEOSTASIS HARMONY

The biphasic changes of the body going from glucose as a primary energy source to a fat based energy source is shown through a cascade of metabolic events. The reader develops an understanding of the human body's adaptability to provide energy from within at the least harm to the body itself.

CHAPTER 6: PROTEIN PUZZLE

The metabolic changes that prevent muscle loss in the obese during dieting are reviewed in detail. The basis of this centers around the adaptation to ketosis (fat breakdown). Muscle strength and endurance can improve even during severe caloric restriction.

CHAPTER 7: GENETIC GRIPE

The heritability of obesity is shown to be due to latent genes that are induced by exposure to environmental factors that then allows their expression.

CHAPTER 8: HORMONES HYPED

Only a rare cause for obesity, hormonal changes are mostly the *result* of weight gain and not the cause; being reversed by weight loss. The new and exciting field of hypothalamic control of appetite by the gut is promising.

CHAPTER 9: MORTALITY MUDDLED

Increased mortality has not been demonstrated for the moderately obese or overweight. It appears that failed attempts at dieting with weight fluctuation are more closely associated with mortality.

CHAPTER 10: POPULAR DIETS DIVULGED

Caloric restriction (eating less) is the major determinant of weight loss rather than the macronutrient (fat, carbohydrate, protein) composition of the diet. Physical activity and dealing with the psychological issues affecting eating behavior are more relevant adaptations than the macronutrients of the diet.

CHAPTER 11: CONCLUSION: TERRIBLE TWO'S

Weight loss is achieved through eating less by changes in eating behavior while weight loss maintenance is much tougher as it is achieved not only by changes in *dietary behavior*, but also, by the addition of *daily exercise* (the terrible two's of maintenance).

Appendix I: From shocking dogs to frightening babies- a theory develops

Appendix II: Children are born with innate fear of water, not food selection

Appendix III: Exercise: the metabolic paradox

Appendix IV: Disease burden of obesity- Stain or Stigma

End Notes

Table of Contents

Introduction

"Nobody dies nowadays of fatal truth; there are too many antidotes to them." *Nietzsche*

In 1980 the prevalence of overweight or obesity among adults age 20 years and older was 47%. In 2002, 2/3 (65%) of the US adult's population (16% of children age 6 to 19) were overweight or obese. The adult is most likely to be a non-Hispanic, African American woman and the child to be a Mexican American boy. Recently, the Surgeon General stated that obesity ranked second only to cigarette smoking as the leading cause of preventable disease and death in the U.S. with a health care cost of approximately 117 billion dollars every year. This obesity epidemic became evident from 1991 to 1998 and exploded across the USA concentrating in the S.E. states. Although the percent of individuals in the overweight class (BMI, Body Mass Index, of 25 to less than 30) has remained relatively stable during the thirty year period, the prevalence of obesity (BMI equal to or more than 30) has increased by more than 50% (from 14.5% to 22.5%).[1]

[1]The BMI is the body weight in kilograms divided by the square of the height in meters. It correlates closely with body fat content outside the normal range (18.5-24.9), and does not account for increase muscle mass of athletes.

According to the USDA Nationwide Food Consumption Survey, the average fat intake in the United States dropped from 41% to 37% of the diet with the average total energy intake decreasing by 3% in women and 6% in men between 1977 and 1988. European studies during the same time period show similar rise in prevalence of obesity with a decline in energy intake. From 1978 to 1991 there has been a fourfold increase in the percent of the US population consuming sugar-substitutes, reduced fat. Also, during this time there was an increase in the consumption of reduced caloric foods from 19 to 76%. With the increased use of reduced-calorie food products and at the same time a reduction in fat and energy intake by western societies, it is evident that these measures have not attenuated the rising prevalence of obesity. Therefore, with reduced dietary intake a substantial decrease in physical activity must be fueling the obesity epidemic. In support of this are studies that show that sedentary individuals are twice as likely to gain substantial weight over a 4-5 year period than physically active men and women. Indeed, 60% of the US adult population report no regular physical activity and 25% report that they are not active at all.

Although 2/3 of American adults are currently overweight or obese, only 1/3 of Americans (37% men and 52% women) see themselves that way. Of those that see themselves as overweight/ obese fewer than 2/3 are trying to lose weight. Among men trying to lose weight, the average weight is 200 pounds with a goal weight of 180 pounds. Among women the average weight is 155 pounds with the goal weight of 130 pounds. Slightly more than 1/3 of normal weight women are trying to lose weight, as compared to 12% of men. Of those trying to lose weight several significant differences were found between 1985 and 1990 in regards to the best ways to lose weight. In 1985 most people thought the best way to lose weight was by "not eating before going to bed" or "by eating fewer calories." "Increasing physical activity" was the third most frequently reported best way to lose weight. In a recent Time/ABC news poll, 86% of Americans feel that "not getting enough physical exercise" and "poor eating habits" are the most important causes of obesity in this country.[2] Although 58% would like to lose weight, only 36% are following a particular diet plan and 26% exercise at least three times per week. Among both sexes tying to lose weight the combination of eating fewer calories and exercising 150 minutes or more per week (the minimal level of physical activity recommended in the national guidelines for all Americans) is reported to be only 1/5.

Trying to maintain weight was reported by about 1/3 of both men and women. About half reported using physical activity as a strategy with 2/3 using diet modification. Slightly more than 1/10 reported the combination of eating fewer calories and exercising 150 minutes or more per week.[3] The National Weight Control Registry is a group of over 3,000 mostly white American women age 45 who have lost at least 30 pounds and maintained that weight loss for more than a year. About half of these Registry individuals report having lost weight on their own without a formal weight loss program through using diet and exercise. On average the majority of participants report eating a low fat, high carbohydrate, low calorie diet with a high level of physical activity. Information gathered from this group would suggest that the optimal amount of exercise to maintain weight loss

[2]Fifty percent of people polled think obesity is caused by genetics.
[3]Among adolescent high school students 44% of the female students and 15% of male students reported that they were trying to loose weight. An additional 26% of female students and 15% of male students reported they were trying to keep from gaining more weight. About 50%of the female students reported exercise and skipping meals as a means of weight control, while 30% of male students use exercise and 18% skip meals to control weight.

is about 1 hour a day of brisk walking or about 2500 to 3000 kcal per week.

With many Americans aware of being overweight/obese, why are they so complacent? This has been brought about by an era of myths surrounding weight loss with little to no attention paid to maintenance of that weight loss. Superimposed on this exist the gray areas in commercial advertising that relate to constitutional protections of free speech, which limit the effective regulation of outlandish claims by some weight loss products. Add to this that many physicians have not received formal training in weight loss and tend to view the obese in terms of society in general as lazy, sad, and lacking in self control. In this regard overweight patients are less likely than those of normal weight to receive adequate health care and often perceive themselves as being treated with distain and disrespect. It is in this atmosphere of outrageous and unsubstantiated claims that overweight/obese individuals are abandoned to make a decision on their own, most often without the true, scientific evidence.

The current myths that dieting and weight loss would cause negative psychological consequences (eating disorders and depression) and severe metabolic disturbances (such as loss of active muscle tissue) come from a study done in 1950 involving normal weight, young men who participated in a semi-starvation experiment in which they ate half of their previous intake for six months. Profound effects were observed across a wide range of functioning. Extreme negative emotions, depression and anger were common. A subgroup of men engaged in binge eating that persisted for a while afterwards. Morphological, biochemical and physiologic changes in a variety of organs including muscle loss were reported. These findings were not unexpected given that their weight was reduced below 25% of normal, meeting the criteria for anorexia nervosa. Findings from this study which present adverse effects of caloric restriction in normal weight individuals are often extrapolated to those who are overweight/obese. This is *not appropriate* as obese individuals seem to be protected from many of these ill effects and a goal of 25% below ideal body weight is not sought. It will be shown that weight loss in the overweight/obese is different from that seen in the lean. If the same processes were occurring during starvation in a lean and obese person, when the lean person died, then the obese one would die still with much of his/her fat stores still present. This obviously does not occur. It is, therefore, to dispel the myths and bring to light the truths of weight loss that this book was written. Through knowledge can these myths and the predators that stalk the obese with disinformation and false claims be exposed.

It was decided not to directly name the many commercial diet pills, exercise programs, and diets that make outlandish claims. It was chosen rather to present the scientific evidence that clearly discredits the basis of their assertions. As discussed in chapter 8, claims that certain hormones are the cause of obesity are dismissed. Most hormonal changes are the result of the excess weight and are reversed with weight loss. In chapter 3, exercise is shown not to produce or add significantly to weight loss without diet. Exercise becomes vital in maintaining the weight loss as a reduced energy state can persist for many years after the initial weight loss (chapter 4). Programs that prey on fears of muscle loss and with that loss of strength are shown to have no significant basis to make that claim in chapters 3 and 6. However, a more direct exposure of the myths of the more popular diets by name was chosen in chapter 10. Finally in appendix IV, mention of a few diet pill ingredients occurs.

Dieting as used in this book refers to the intentional and sustained restriction of caloric intake for the purpose of reducing body weight.

The restriction of caloric intake has at its extreme starvation, which is not considered dieting but is brought to attention for purposes of delineating certain facts that occur with weight loss. Because dietary restriction in children and adolescents poses special concerns, the conclusions derived from this review should be considered applicable to adults only. Almost all of the studies sited are with adult's age 20 or greater.

PROLOGUE

Allison B. was a patient for many years before she had to change doctors as I was no longer on her insurance preferred provider list. I continued to see her husband, Bob, who has a different insurance. It is through Bob that I have come to have Allison's diary. For several months after Allison decided to have gastric bypass for the treatment of her obesity, she had a rocky recovery. She seemed to be in the hospital more than out of it. She had a blood clot to her lung (pulmonary embolus) shortly after her third surgery for small bowel obstruction and died suddenly at the age of 42. Allison had kept a diary for the year before her gastric bypass. Her husband found it and one day brought it to me in the hope that I could use it to help others. Bob had read it over and over and he insisted the diary was basically Allison's daily struggle with weight. Since Bob knew I had a special interest in weight loss, he thought the diary would give me insight into the mind of someone desperate to lose weight. I tried not to take it but at his insistence I accepted it on the premise of putting it on a shelf for safe keeping if ever he wanted it back. Some years later I came across the diary and it caught my attention. Bob had been right. Allison's diary, that is her life, had been focused on her daily struggle to loose weight. What was more important was the fact that she had been misled by the myths that have evolved around weight loss. These myths blocked her attempts time and time again. She was, and is not, alone.

So much disinformation about weight loss is pervasive that many Americans are confounded into complacency. Not only patients but most doctors, nurses and other health care professionals are poorly informed. Most of the current medical dogma of weight loss comes from studies that didn't involve obese individuals and were of too short of duration. Yet, scientific facts (many are decades old) that have shattered this wall of ignorance have not been brought to light. It is for this purpose that I write this book: to expose the myths that have wrapped themselves around the large body of scientific evidence deceiving many from achieving and maintaining weight loss. I have taken a passage from the diary and then exposed a myth using evidence from scientific studies. It is hoped that through this knowledge we can throw off the myths that have prevented us as a society to shed the burdens of obesity.

Chapter 1
Psychological Passions

Diary Entry September 3rd

My psychiatrist asked me to keep a diary. He may has well have asked me to keep a food diary. My whole life is built around food. Last weekend Bob and I got into a fight about if we were going to eat before or after the movie. I don't know why because we ate before during and after the movie. After work all I can think of is what I am going to eat when I get home. I have had to hide the potato chips from Bob so I can have a few (let's not kid ourselves the whole bag). I cannot seem to stop eating once I start and then I feel guilty about the amount I have eaten. It's my reward for making it through the day. My psychiatrist wants to know why I am so depressed; the reason faces me every morning getting dressed. I am ashamed of my body and it's depressing. While at work I get dumped on with extra work while that skinny bimbo gets to go out to lunch with the boss and she gets the promotion. My psychiatrist says that shame is like a mushroom, it grows in the dark on dead decomposing material. When brought out to the light it withers. So if I can expose my shame it will go away. Why would I want to expose my body when even I don't like to see it?

Diary entry September 7th

I came home and found my daughter having sex with her boyfriend in my living room. He is at least twice her age. This has brought back some bad memories, particularly that regarding uncle Willie. When Dad was off to War uncle Willie would come over and touch me in bad places. I know now that he sexually abused me. When Dad did come home and I told him, he took a stick to me calling me all kinds of names as if it were my fault. I obviously grew up in a dysfunctional family, who doesn't? I always was in constant fear of being abandoned, but they always provided a roof and food on the table. I guess it was their way of showing me that they really loved me. My third husband would say to me that I could not deal with kindness but I got years of learning how to deal with abuse. My psychiatrist says that I substitute food for loneliness and over the years it has gotten easier to do so.

Diary entry September 15th

I have decided to lose weight. I am really committed this time. Today I bent over to pick up an M&M that dropped out of my drawer at work and I split my pants right down the middle. I used safety pins to put it together. I forgot about it and when I tried to deliver papers to the City Hall I couldn't get past the metal detector. The metal detector kept going off over my butt. I bet they thought "This lady needs to get the lead out of her ass."

Diary entry September 17th

Funny how everyone around me is trying to destroy my diet. When I lost before, I remember feeling better about myself, however that seemed to cause others to be concerned. Bob, although I love him dearly, is not a prime catch. I know I settled for him. I am sure he stopped taking me out when I was thin because of the looks other men gave me. I am sure that he felt threatened. He didn't realize how vulnerable this made me feel. I know that my fat friends were jealous telling me to go exercise in the thin class which we used to refer to as the bimbo group. I remember how Lucy no longer would talk to me because I was no longer her "fat friend". I am sure I made her feel good about herself when I was the fat one.

Diary entry September 28th

I look at my friend's young children and wonder how they can eat the way they do and not get fat. I have been told by my pediatrician many years ago that children have an innate ability to instinctively select and consume a well balanced diet. So what happens to this when we grow up? How do we lose that ability?

This scenario presents many of the psychological aspects of obesity. The psychology of obesity and weight loss over the past 40 years has centered around whether psychological disease caused or was the result of obesity. As a result, psychiatry got stuck on trying to decide whether the chicken came before the egg or not. The field of obesity psychology stagnated for a long time. Weight loss has been shown to improve self esteem and overall well-being. So why do so many people overeat and continue to do so when the consequences are so negative?[1] To make things worse, the advertising media has had a significant adverse impact of reinforcing a pattern of overeating. As the food environment has changed to increase food availability, there has, also, been a dramatic increase in exposure to messages that encourage food consumption through television. Exposure to food advertising especially commercials for fast food or convenient foods seems to influence the viewer's food choices toward higher fat or higher energy foods. Television has been sited as a contributing factor to higher dietary energy and fat intake. Television is the most widely used advertising media, which is not surprising given that televisions are present in 98% of U.S. households and adults spend an average of 2 hours a day watching television. Obviously, the associated diseases and physical discomfort of being obese are not desirable. Yet relapse is high. Why? The etiology of obesity must be understood in order to understand its impact in weight loss.

Obesity, for the most part, is the result of learned helplessness to social pressures and it's because these are not addressed, relapse is high (see appendix I for a more detailed discussion of learned helplessness). Therefore, the psychological processes that lead to obesity overwhelm the physical needs of the body. This mal-adaptive behavioral pattern of over eating has it roots in "disinhitition", which is the loss of control following a cognitive, emotional or

---

[1]After a minimum of 100 pound weight loss in patients undergoing surgery, these reduced obese people were asked to choose between being obese again or being deaf, diabetic, blind or amputee. No one chose obesity. All viewed only blindness and amputation as being worse than obesity.

pharmacological event. This loss of control produces anxiety that results in a sense of shame.

The most common pattern of eating in the overweight and obese is referred to as binge eating. This is present in 20 to 50% of obese patient's seeking treatment, where as only 2% of a community sample has this eating disorder. Binge eating disorder (BED) is defined as eating a large amount of food with a sense of lack of control followed by feelings of guilt over how much was eaten, usually occurring at least twice a week, and not engaging in compensatory purging such as vomiting or use of laxatives. The incident of BED increases with the severity of obesity and is associated with early onset of obesity, frequent weight cycling (yo-yo), body shape disparagement, and psychological problems. Even among obese non-bingers with depression, those with BED have significantly more problems with mood or depression.

Negative moods such as sadness, anger or boredom often precede a binge episode and are almost always followed by feelings of guilt. It is well known that individuals with BED, undergoing weight loss treatment will have less weight loss and larger lapses in adherence and weight re-gain than similarly treated obese non-binge eaters. Furthermore, there is little scientific evidence for carbohydrate craving (chocolate) during binge eating. In fact, fats appear to be the preferential food choice. In regards to individuals presenting with an inability to lose weight despite a history of caloric restriction (reduced food intake), there is evidence that this is due to severely misreporting their food intake and level of physical activity and is not due to an abnormality in metabolism. This means that many obese individuals are caught up in a denial state.[2]

Although binge eaters are more likely to have weight cycling (yo-yo) it is not apparent that weight cycling is the cause of binge eating, nor does it cause psychological problems. Numerous studies during the past thirty years have reported reductions in symptoms of depression and anxiety but no worsening in affect or mood in obese patients treated by behavior modification combined with moderate or severe caloric restriction with or without weight loss medications. Neither the number of diets attempted or the total lifetime weight loss/gain cycles are related to the development of depression. A history of weight cycling has not been related to other long term adverse psychological effects. Those obese or overweight people who lost weight and maintained that weight loss for more than three years report improvement in their overall quality of life, level of energy, mobility, general mood and self confidence as seen in Table 1.1, which is a survey of thousands of obese individuals who have lost weight and been able to maintain that weight loss.

Nonetheless, the disinhibited (loss of control) eating pattern of obese individuals has its roots in emotional disturbances. The etiological significance of sadness, anger and boredom must be addressed for successful weight loss and maintenance to occur. Although this forms the basis for the etiology of obesity, other

---

[2]There are three stages which an individual experiences grief and they follow a predictable sequence. First, there is denial, followed by anger, then attempts at resolution. For example, a person is told he/she has lung cancer. First there is denial in that it could not be happening to them and request more testing or a 2nd opinion is sought. Then anger is expressed as why me, why not the neighbor down the street who smoked 3 packs/day? Then begins acceptance. I have seen people progress through these stages over a matter of minutes, while others get hung up in one stage for years. But, for grief to resolve, all stages must be experienced.

Table1.1 Effect of weight loss on other areas of life[a]

Determinant	Improved	No difference	Worse
Quality of life	95.3	4.3	0.4
Level of energy	92.4	6.7	0.9
Mobility	92.3	7.1	0.6
General mood	91.4	6.9	1.6
Self-confidence	90.9	9.0	0.1
Physical health	85.8	12.9	1.3
Interactions with			
opposite sex	65.2	32.9	0.9
same sex	50.2	46.8	0.4
strangers	69.5	30.4	0.1
Time spent interacting with			
others	59.1	39.6	1.3
Job performance	54.5	45.0	0.6
Other hobbies	49.1	36.7	0.4
Interactions with			
parents	32.8	65.0	2.2
Interactions with			
spouse	56.3	37.3	5.9
Time spent thinking about			
food	49.1	36.7	14.2
weight	51.0	28.6	20.4

[a]$N = 784$. Results indicate percentage.

Wing, RenaR. and Hill, James O. (2001). Successful weight loss maintenance. *Annu Rev Nutr*,21,323-41.Reprinted with permission from the Annual Review of Nutrition, volume 21©2001 by Annual Reviews www.annualreviews.org.

problems are triggered as a result of weight loss that, also, need to be evaluated and treated if success is to occur.

These problems that evolve as a result of weight loss occur in three areas: the self, socialization and skills acquisition.

Weight loss can cause increased feelings of vulnerability, insecurity and the uncovering of weaknesses that can no longer be blamed on obesity. Many female weight loss patients have reported an increase sense of vulnerability and being viewed as sexual by men. They felt the excess weight had protected them from fearful sexual advances. This fear of sexual vulnerability may have its roots in sexual abuse. One out of every four obese patients presenting to a weight loss clinic in San Diego in 1993 acknowledged sexual abuse during infancy, childhood or adolescents, compared to only 6% of the always slender group used for comparison.[3] Of these obese patients 22% were conscious of using obesity to reduce sexual fears, (for example to minimize sexual attractiveness to decrease spousal jealousy).

Often many of the activities that were associated with the old friend are no longer conducive to the reduced one's new lifestyle. Weight loss can have a destabilizing effect on some marriages and intimate relationships. As individuals lose weight, self-esteem improves and many weight reduced individuals report conflicts with old friends, frequently due to jealousy and insecurity on the part of the old friend, in which the reduced person is no longer the "fat friend" that often made the old friend feel better. Mood and activeness increase and dependence on the other partner diminishes. Desire for more autonomy by the reduced-obese individual can result in

---

[3]Of the sexual abuse voiced by obese patients 13% was by incest, 9% molestation by someone outside of the family and 3% by forceful rape by a non-relative. Of these 29% had a subsequent abuse experience. 4% of obese patients "did not recall" but none of the always slender were uncertain of recall.

insecurity and fear of abandonment by the other partner. Conflict of emotion can occur with weight loss. For some there is a struggle with resentment and anger at being treated better than when they were obese and this can spill over into a feeling of suspiciousness. The "emotional eaters" have the most difficulty adapting to the situation. They have the added challenge of having to find alternative means of coping with negative emotions. Furthermore, development of new social skills and skills of negotiation have to be developed. Weight-reduced individuals must impose a change in their lifestyle of eating and exercise in order to cope with these self-esteem and social pressures. Many lack the social skills to adapt to their new lifestyle and find it easier to relapse back to obesity in order to cope in ways that have become familiar.

For the post gastric bypass patient the dramatic change in their eating behavior is forced on them with the consequence of any deviation from the strict diet would most likely result in the adverse "dumping syndrome".[4] Later these patients start increasing the amount of food eaten so as not to induce the dumping syndrome. Their stomachs stretch to have increased capacity and with that the dumping stops. Without the adverse effects of dumping, a pattern of disinhibited (loss of control) eating redevelops. With the majority of these patients a daily conscious effort to diet has to be established, reminiscence of failed dieting attempts in the past.[5] This explains why

---

[4]Dumping Syndrome refers to the symptoms that occur after a meal in which the contents of that meal has very little or no time in the stomach and are "dumped" into the small intestine. This rapid emptying of particles into the small intestine draws fluid into the lumen as would occur if one were to place water next to a small pile of sugar on the table (osmotic pressure). This fluid shift into the gut produces acute distension and a drop in the blood volume from where the water is drawn. This produces pain, nausea, sweating and light headedness.

the greatest weight loss occurs in the first year after the operation and the weight averages only 35% loss of initial body weight.

Most obese individuals are likely to have grown up in a family that did not provide stability and emotional support during childhood. Parental loss, parental alcoholism, or abuse (sexual or mental) are common in the obese who report increased depression and anxiety. Childhood attempts to cope with these stresses usually involve eating as a means of gratification. In *People magazine* Oprah Winfrey summed it up as: "My greatest failure was in believing that the weight issue was about weight. It's not. It's about not handling stress properly. It's about sexual abuse. It's about all the things that cause other people to become alcoholics, or drug addicts".

Allison brings up an interesting topic in her last entry regarding children. This topic is perhaps the most misunderstood, misinterpreted topic in obesity. Since this book is dealing primarily with adult weight loss I would refer the reader to Appendix II to review the topic of childhood diet selection.

---

[5]This daily conscious effort is referred to as "restrained eating". These individuals constantly restrain from overeating through various methodologies of avoiding certain food groups or counting calories.

Chapter 2
Metabolic Mysteries

Diary entry October 17th

Every time I diet I seem to lose weight for the first two weeks. After which I hit this plateau. Even though I am eating the same thing that I ate two weeks ago I am no longer losing weight. I just don't understand it. I tried to exercise harder but I am more fatigued. If I skip a day of exercise or I eat a few more calories one day it seems the next day I have a weight gain. This does not seem to happen unless I am trying to loose weight. I can be my regular old fat self eat a few extra calories one day or not exercise for a week and not gain weight.

For overweight people to lose weight there must be a reduction of energy intake. The measure of energy in food is the caloric content of that food expressed as so many calories (cal or kcal) per portion. Therefore, a reduction in calories is a necessary requirement for weight reduction. Often obese individuals who wish to lose weight find their efforts thwarted. They are faced with the fact that the body has evolved a number of effective responses which are designed to maintain the current weight. These physiological responses regulate body weight by adapting to the difference between energy intake and energy output by the body, so that a decrease in energy intake is met with a decrease in energy utilization. These responses form the metabolic adaptation to reduced energy intake (dieting) that oppose weight loss.[1] These compensatory responses that reduce energy utilization often frustrate the efforts at achieving and maintaining weight loss.

Energy that is consumed is utilized by the body for cellular function, cardiopulmonary activity, digestion and physical activity. All these require energy and result in heat production. The Total Energy Expenditure (24 hour TEE) of the body is broken down into three components. Approximately 60% of the 24 hour TEE is the metabolic cost of processes involved in cellular and cardiopulmonary activity and is referred to as the **Resting** or **Basal Metabolic Rate** (RMR or BMR).[2] The energy or heat expended in digestion, transport, and deposition of nutrients accounts for about 10% of the 24 hour TEE and is the **Thermic Effect of Food (TEF)**.[3] Physical activity accounts for the remaining 30% of the 24 hour TEE. Often the TEF and the heat lost during physical activity are separately referred to

---

[1]These responses evolved early in humans, allowing for survival during famine. It appears that certain groups of humans evolved more efficient responses, thereby creating a diversity of weight changes by different individuals on the same diet. This is discussed in more detail in chapter 7.

[2]BMR is the minimum rate of energy expenditure immediately on awakening from sleep, having abstained from food and heavy exercise for at least 12 hours and obtained while supine. In contrast, the RMR is determined sitting or prone at least 4 hours after light activity or a light meal at anytime during the day.

[3]Eating increases the metabolic rate immediately by the TEF for 1.5 to 8 hours following a meal. There is a second component that occurs with overfeeding and lasts for several days.

as the "**Non-R**esting Energy Expenditure" (NREE) as compared to the RMR. See figure 2.0.

Measurement of the energy expenditure is frequently done by two methods. The first method is based on the fact that oxygen consumption and carbon dioxide production occur at different rates during the combustion (utilization for energy) of carbohydrate, protein, fat and alcohol. Using a facemask, mouthpiece, canopy or chamber, these gases are collected and using equations the metabolic rate can be measured using this indirect calorimeter method. Metabolic rates for the RMR, TEF and physical activity are usually measured this way. By the second method, the 24 hour TEE is often measured over one to two weeks using injection of small amounts of heavy water (H_2"**O**")and measuring the rate of carbon dioxide made from that different form of "**O**"$_2$ (C"**O**"$_2$))

Fat is not considered very metabolically active so RMR is thought to be mainly due to the **Fat Free Mass** (FFM or lean body mass) of the body representing mostly muscle, but also other organs of the body. RMR is very different between individuals (plus or minus 25%) but is consistent within the same individual (plus or minus 5%). Components of the RMR contribute at different rates in that skeletal muscle, which constitutes about 43% of the total mass in an adult, contributes only 22 to 36% of the RMR, whereas, the brain, which is only about 2% of the body mass, contributes 20 to 24% of the RMR. Other factors affect the RMR. The RMR declines with age, is higher in men and can differ between different families as well as ethnic group. As noted in footnote 3, overfeeding enhances RMR within 24 hours, however underfeeding requires several days before a progressive lowering effect is seen.

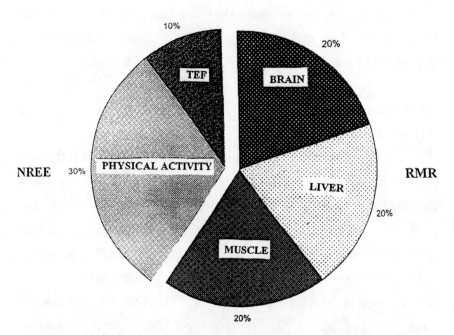

24 HOUR TEE

Fig. 2.0 The 24 hour Total Energy Expenditure(**24hrTEE**) can be divided into the Resting Metabolic Rate(**RMR**) and the Non-Resting Energy Expenditure(**NREE**).The brain, liver, and muscle contribute about equally to the RMR, which is about 60% of the 24hrTEE. The remaining 40% is composed of the Thermic Effect of Food(**TEF**) and the physical activity expenditure.

FFM can be measured by many methods: *hydrostatic weighing* is based on the fact that fat is less dense than FFM, so fat people displace less water; *total body water* assumes that fat contains no water and all water exists in lean tissue in a constant proportion; *total body potassium* method uses a similar constant in that 98% of potassium in the body is in the lean tissue. Therefore, by measuring potassium or water content we are measuring FFM. Other means of measurement include: *Anthropometric* (the size of body parts) measurements; the *Body Mass Index* (BMI) using measurements of height, weight and sex; and, other methods using *electrical conductivity impendence, neutron activation of nitrogen, CT scanning,* etc. Using these methods, a 70kg (154 pounds) non-obese man averages 20% fat and 80% lean (FFM) tissue. By itself, lean tissue consists of 73% water, 20% protein, 5% minerals, and 1% Glycogen.

Excess weight in obese people is about 75% fat and 25% FFM. Since RMR is associated with the metabolically active FFM, any change in one would represent a similar change in the other. Therefore, obese people with their excess weight have an increased FFM and, therefore, a higher metabolic rate than non-obese individuals. See figure 2.1. Yet, in the 1970's obese people were believed to have a dietary intake no higher and an activity level no less than lean people, and their inability to lose weight was felt to be due to a low metabolic rate. However, no evidence of an energy sparing metabolic state has been found in healthy, obese individuals who are at stable weight. On the other hand, it is well established that weight loss is accompanied by loss of this excess FFM (weight loss composition is similar to composition of excessive weight gained: 75% fat and 25% FFM), and therefore, a decline in the RMR and as well as a decline in the 24 hour TEE. However, the reduction in the FFM, or RMR, could not account for the total reduction in the 24 hour TEE. Therefore,

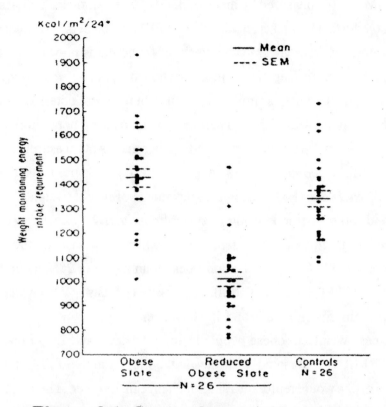

Figure 2.1 Seven-day weight maintaining energy intake requirements, or 24-hr TEE, in 26 subjects(12 males and 14 females) studied when obese and after substantial weight loss(reduced-obese state) in comparison to requirements of 26 never-obese, normal-weight subjects(controls) matched by sex and age. Although the reduced-obese averaged 220 lbs *vs* 137 lbs for controls, the reduced-obese had a 28% reduction in energy requirement compared to their obese state and required 25% less than their lighter controls. Leibel, Rudolph L. and Hirsch, Jules. (1984). Diminished energy requirements in reduced-obese patients. *Metabolism*, 33(2),164-170. Reprinted with permission from Elsevier, copyright 1984.

something else had to be occurring to add to the drop the 24-hr TEE besides the loss of FFM and in the 1980's obesity research was obsessed at finding an answer to this dilemma.

In a 1986 study male and female, obese individuals had their jaws wired closed and placed on 2 pints of skimmed milk/day for 90 to 250 days to obtain an average 26% reduction in weight. The 24 hour TEE dropped on average 25% lower than predicted for the new, reduced weight achieved. Although the fall in RMR was closely related to the fall in FFM, or muscle, half of the decrease in the total 24 hour TEE could not be explained by the fall in RMR alone. There had to be a reduction in the non-resting energy expenditure (NREE) consisting of the thermic effect of food and physical activity (See figure 2.2, refresh yourself on the components of the 24-hr TEE from fig. 2.0). The fact that the decline in the 24 hour TEE with weight loss was found to occur mainly during the day and not at night would suggest that the reduction in NREE was indeed part of this disproportionately, reduced metabolic state of weight loss, since people are more active during the day than while sleeping. In fact the NREE was found to be lower per a given amount of FFM during weight loss as compared to stable weight FFM, unlike the RMR which was proportional to the drop in FFM. Because the thermic effect of food is relatively constant (10% of ingested calories), then a reduction in physical activity energy would be the determining factor in the reduction of the NREE. Even when there was an increase in exercise done at training levels of sufficient intensity to substantially increase work capacity, the diet-induced reduction of the total metabolic rate was not reversed and was no different from those who did not exercise. Also, it was noted that the RMR consistently returned to pre-exercise levels within 1 hour after stopping exercise. Therefore, exercise would have little

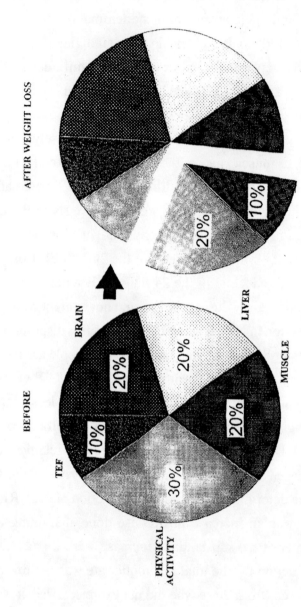

24 hr TEE

BEFORE

TEF 10%
BRAIN 20%
PHYSICAL ACTIVITY 30%
MUSCLE 20%
20%

AFTER WEIGHT LOSS

20%
LIVER 10%

Fig. 2.2 The effect of weight loss on the 24hr TEE. There is a 20% decrease in the RMR mostly from the FFM, or muscle component, which represents about a 10% decrease in the total 24hr TEE. (Since the RMR is 60% of the 24hr TEE, a 20% drop would be 20% of 60%, or about 10%, of the total.) But, there is a total drop in the 24hr TEE of 30%. This would mean that there is a 20% drop in the physical activity energy component (the TEF remains fairly constant) which represents 2/3, or roughly 70%, of the total 30% decrease in the 24hr TEE.

holdover effect on the RMR in any event. Even the RMR per unit of fat free mass (muscle) was found not to be augmented by training exercise during weight loss. In fact the drop in RMR with weight loss is independent of body composition, aerobic fitness, and not affected by whether a severely restricted diet (782 kcal/day) or a moderately restricted diet (1369 kcal/day) is followed. The deeper the scientists looked into this discrepancy the more elusive the answer became.

The adult brain which is mostly lipids consumes 20% of the RMR. The liver which consumes another 20% of the RMR is involved in making glucose and ketones as fuel for the brain. Adipose tissue is relatively inert consuming 2-5%. Muscle consumes additional 20% of the RMR and is involved in protein synthesis and thereby might be a regulator of energy expenditure. However, protein synthesis does not change with weight loss and, therefore, is not a significant contributor to the disproportional reduction in the 24 hour TEE seen with weight loss. Those dieters that frequently regained (yoyo) were not found to have a more efficient metabolism than non-yoyo dieters, nor was fat distribution a factor in whether one yoyo'ed or not. The length of time that someone had been obese was not shown to have an effect on the rate of decline in RMR or weight loss. Furthermore, age and regional fat distribution (hip vs abdominal) have no effect on the reduction of RMR with weight loss. However, these studies found a sustained decrease in RMR accompanying weight loss that persisted for years despite increased caloric intake and weight stabilization.

The central finding in these early studies is that there is a sharp decline in total weight *maintenance* energy requirements that accompany weight reduction in obese individuals. See figure 2.1. Obese subjects that have lost at least 10% of their original weight have on the average a 15%to 25% decrease in the RMR, but a 30% decrease in 24 hour TEE as compared to others at the same weight who have not lost weight. The reduction in the 24 hour TEE of reduced obese individuals is usually 25% lower than predicted by the reduction of FFM observed, and therefore, the reduction in the 24 hour TEE cannot be fully explained by the reduction of lean tissue (FFM) or RMR alone. As we have seen the 24 hour TEE can be broken down into three components. The reduced RMR accounts for 25 to 30% of the total 24 hour TEE decline as accounted for by the loss of FFM. Therefore, the thermic effect of food (TEF) and the thermic effect of exercise, which compromise the non-resting energy expenditure account for the majority (70%) of the 24 hour TEE reduction. Since TEF is relatively small and appears relatively constant (about 10% of ingested calories), the major reduction in total energy requirements is, therefore, attributable to the reduction in physical activity related energy expenditure, and has been shown to account for 70% of the decrease in 24-hour TEE with the remaining 25-30% accounted for by the proportional decrease in FFM or RMR. See figure 2.2. Reduced exercise-related energy expenditure (non-resting energy expenditure, NREE) of formerly obese people may be due not only to lower body weight but due to changes in the efficiency with which skeletal muscle converts chemical energy to mechanical energy or by some other unknown metabolic process. Furthermore, when compared to normal weight people the reduced work of movement accompanying weight loss cannot entirely explain the enhanced metabolic efficiency of reduced-obese people since in most studies on the average the reduced-obese are still much heavier (by 81 pounds in one study) than people who have never lost weight. Even when the reduced-obese obtained and stabilized at ideal body weight, they had about a 15% -25% lower metabolic rate than those at the same weight who had never loss weight at all levels of activity.

In conclusion, studies of obese individuals show that a reduction of 10% or more in body weight is associated with a compensatory drop in the total energy expenditure that tends to oppose the weight loss. Furthermore, these compensatory changes can persist for four to six years after the initial weight loss has stabilized, in which lower needs of energy intake are required to maintain that new weight than others at the same weight who have not lost weight. After weight loss this reduction in energy requirement to maintain body function and activity is estimated to be on average 375 to 500 calories per day.[4] Thus, the reduced individual must overcome this energy savings by an increase in exercise related activity on the order of 440 calories per day. This would be adding a time of walking at 3 miles per hour for 100 minutes per day if no restriction of food intake is made. This is comparable to data from the National Weight Control Registry of over 3,000 subjects who have lost at least 30 pounds and maintained that weight loss for an average of six years. In that group the women average about 320 calories per day of exercise and the men average 470 calories per day of exercise.

The implication of these findings is that a significant increase in exercise-related energy expenditure (on the order of 500 kcal/day for a 20% weight loss) is needed to overcome the decreased energy needs

---

[4]The average daily intake of the US adult is around 2500 cal/day. If the energy reduction is 15% that would result in a 375 cal/day reduction, a 20% energy reduction would result in a 500 cal/day reduction. Compare this to the current exercise recommendations for a 200 lb. person in chapter 3. Exercise that is recommended for one week for never obese individuals would be needed daily by the reduced-obese.

(reduced 24-hr TEE) of the reduced-obese.[5] To compensate for this decreased metabolic state, the reduced obese must add or recruit more active lean tissue. Therefore, individuals that have lost weight must exercise more as compared to those who are at the same weight who have never lost weight. As one would imagine this would predispose weight reduced individuals to regaining the weight lost (yo-yoing) if exercise is not incorporated into their maintenance program. In the past this has given raise to the concept of a *set point* in that there is a genetic pre-disposition to maintain or return (Yo-Yo) to a certain body composition for weight. However, individuals undergoing gastric bypass from one institute have maintained a 55% weight reduction after 14 years. This would argue against the *set point*. Nonetheless, there appears to be a metabolic "memory" that persists for at least six years following weight reduction against which the reduced obese individual must continue to struggle. This struggle must overcome the reduced exercise-related energy expenditure by incorporating daily exercise.

---

[5]The only exception to this rule is the finding that RMR remains normal following Roux-en-Y gastric bypass (RYGB) despite intake comparable to a very low caloric diet. Although vertical banded gastroplasty (VGB) causes a similar low intake, the decline in RMR is similar to that of diet restriction. The only major anatomic difference between RYGB and VBG is the bypass of the first part of the small intestine. Therefore, the mechanism for the maintenance of a normal RMR with RYGB must be mediated by alterations in the secretion of gut peptides that influence the hypothalamus of the brain. See chapter 8 for more details of these hormones.

Chapter 3
Exercise Escapades

Diary entry November 18th

It has been four weeks and the scales say I have not lost weight. I must be changing fat into muscle with the exercise class. I am more and more tired, but I must increase my exercise to raise my metabolism and burn more calories if I am to continue losing.

This scenario represents one the most common myths about weight loss. Many scientific studies demonstrate that an overweight or obese individual's exercise does not contribute significantly to weight reduction. Nonetheless, consumers spent 4.8 billion dollars on home exercise equipment in 1996, more than 100% increased from 1990. Over 50% of all U.S. adults own some kind of home exercise equipment. Home exercise equipment is used at least once a week in 65% of households that own the equipment. Between 1988 and 1998 health club membership grew 51% and it is interesting that this "boom" in health club membership occurred during the same time striking increases in weight gain in the population in general were observed. On the average 1 pound of body fat stores about 3,500 calories of energy. A 75kg (165pounds) person utilizes approximately 100 calories to walk one mile. That person would have to walk about 35 miles to expend the amount of energy contained in one pound of fat. For individuals who need to lose 44 to 60 pounds of fat, it is obviously a formidable challenge to lose that much by exercise. The surgeon general and the AMA recommend that individuals should perform at least 30 minutes of moderately intense physical exercise on most days of the week in order to improve health and lose weight. This would mean that a 200 pound person walking a brisk four miles per hour would burn 147 calories per 30 minute session. Exercising four times a week (most days) would total 588 calories per week, thereby losing slightly less than one pound per month. If this person worked up to an hour a day four times a week, the weight loss would be a little over 2 pounds a month.

Although exercise alone promotes weight loss, the amount of weight that can be lost quickly is less than that achieved through dieting alone. Therefore, many studies were done in the 1980's to see if the addition of exercise to reduction diets would accelerate weight loss. However, many studies found that adding exercise to a calorie-restricted diet did not increase significantly the amount of weight lost. Furthermore, exercise added to diet did not increase the loss of weight as fat for men (70% for diet alone vs 69% for diet plus exercise) or for women (89% for diet alone vs 79%). Even when the intensity of exercise was varied from 80-90% to 40-50% of maximal effort, there was no difference between the two in weight loss or fat loss.

Figure 3.1 is a good study that summaries what many studies demonstrated singularly: that exercise does not contribute significantly to weight reduction in overweight/obese individuals. A closer look at this graph reveals many interesting observations. The subjects were overweight women placed on a very low calorie diet (405/kcal/per day) for eight weeks followed by a maintenance diet of 1,500 calories per day while their weight stabilized. The bike exercise consisted of three 20 minute sessions per week at 8.4 miles per hour. Weight exercise was undertaken using a universal machine and six positions involving arms and legs. The cross over group undertook first diet with bike exercise for six weeks then followed by eight weeks of weight training. The groups that only exercised either aerobically with biking or with isotonic resistance (weight training) had no weight loss or a slight gain in weight, respectfully. The groups that undertook diet alone or with exercise achieved and maintained weight loss in similar patterns. This graph clearly deflates the popular myth that exercise helps to reduce body weight and particularly that building muscle produces weight loss. Another fact is that aerobic and isotonic resistance training can be undertaken and sustained during periods of weight reduction while on a very low calorie diet. Furthermore, the diet plus isotonic training groups had a significant improvement in strength per body weight. Dieting subjects showed no deterioration of strength by completion of the diet and dieting subjects performing aerobic training obtained a small additional improvement in aerobic capacity, or the length of time it takes to build up lactic acid to produce aching muscles. This suggests that the weight loss during severe caloric restriction of a very low calorie diet of 5 weeks does not affect muscle efficiency in overweight individuals.

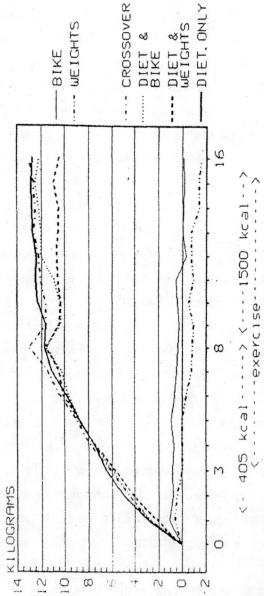

Fig. 3.1 Cumulative weekly weight loss during 8 weeks of diet(405 kcal/day) and 8 weeks of maintenance(1500 kcal/day) with various types of exercise vs diet only. The negative numbers are for weight gain as seen with biking(three 20 minute periods per week at 8.4 mph) and weights(3 times a week doing 3 times 10 repetitions at 60-70% maximum lift). The crossover group did diet and 6 weeks bike followed by 8 week weights. Reprinted by permission from Macmillian Publishers Ltd:Lemons, AD, Kreitzman, SN, Coxon, A, and Howard, A. (1989) Selection of appropriate exercise regimes for weight reduction during vlcd and maintenance. *International J of Obesity*, 13 (suppl.2), 119-123. Copyright 1989

In a study of both men and women placed on a very low calorie diet, those that exercised 6 times a day, 6 days a week, at 50% of their maximal capacity for 10-20 minutes each time had no significant increase in weight loss as compared to those who did not exercise. Although there was evidence of increased utilization of fat during and following exercise, the ratio of fat loss to weight loss was the same in both groups.[1] Nonetheless, the exercise group developed a considerable increased work capacity.

As discussed in Chapter 2, excess weight gained or lost in obese individuals is about 75% fat and 25% fat free mass (FFM), or lean tissue. So weight loss is associated with the loss of FFM (lean body weight) which is metabolically very active producing some 60% of total energy expenditure of the body. This is expressed as the basal metabolic weight (BMR) or resting metabolic rate (RMR) and reduction of RMR seen with weight loss is due in part to this loss of FFM. In Figure 3.2 one can see that the exercise only group (resistance weight training) increased weight; however, when exercise is added to a diet reduced by 1,000 calories per day, lean body mass (FFM) is preserved, although the diet induced total body weight loss was unaffected. However, this preservation of FFM during weight loss with exercise is not associated with any statistically significant reduction in the decline in the RMR seen in weight loss as shown in Table 3.1 that combines results of many other studies on this topic. When obese women are placed on a more severe diet of a five week program of 800 kcal per day, exercise during caloric restricted weight loss did not prevent the drop in RMR even with preservation of protein stores, and the decline in exercising subjects was not different

[1]When fat is utilized for energy there is an increase in its breakdown products of fatty acids and glycerol in the blood and a lowering of the Respiratory Quotient (RQ, which is discussed in chapter 7). This paradox of exercise not adding to weight loss is further discussed in appendix III.

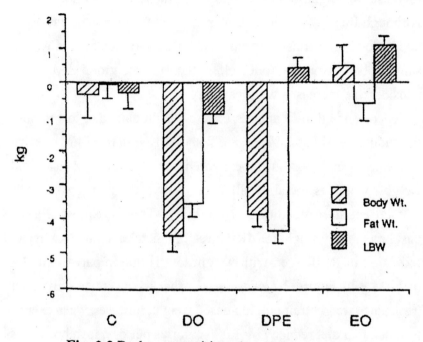

Fig. 3.2 Body composition changes as a result of diet and exercise(resistance weight training) intervention. LBW= lean body weight, C= control(no diet or routine exercise), DO= diet only, DPE= diet plus exercise, EO= exercise only. Adding weight training did not increase the rate of weight loss for the DPE group, but gains were noted in LBW. Ballor, Douglas L., et al. (1988). Resistance weight training during caloric restriction enhances lean body weight maintenance. *Am J Clin Nutr*, 47, 19-25.Permission granted by the American Society for Nutrition, copyright 1988.

	Men	Women	Marginal mean
DO	− 0.63 (0.21) [− 11%]	− 0.54 (0.04) [− 12%]	− 0.59 (0.04)
DPE	− 0.75 (0.42) [− 13%]	− 0.54 (0.08) [− 12%]	− 0.59 (0.13)
Marginal mean	− 0.71 (0.21)	− 0.54 (0.04)	− 0.59 (0.04)

Table 3.1 Changes in resting metabolic rate(RMR)following interventions of exercise training and/or dietary restriction from 60 different study groups of 650 subjects of at least 4 weeks duration. DO=diet only, DPE= diet plus exercise, and marginal mean indicating no significant difference with exercise intervention. Since the % decline in the RMR is not significantly different, there appears to be no exercise benefit to weight loss in regards to changing the metabolic rate. Ballor, Douglas L. and Eric T. Poehlman. (1995). A meta-analysis of the effects of exercise and/dietary restriction on resting metabolic rate. *Eur J Appl Physiol*, 71, 535-542. With the kind permission of Springer Science and Business Media, copyright 1995.

from the decline in non-exercisers. Therefore, exercise programs that promote weight loss through raising metabolism have no scientific basis to make that claim. It is not clear why dietary restriction would block improvement in RMR, unlike non-weight loss exercisers. After all, several studies support a slight improvement in RMR after exercise training in non-weight loss subjects. At present it is not known what tissues contribute to any increase in RMR produced by single or repeated bouts of exercise training in non-weight loss individuals.[2]

Therefore, there must be a compensatory mechanism which attenuates the effect of exercise during weight loss. As show in figure 3.3, in women consuming a 500 calorie per day diet, there were post exercise reductions in oxygen consumption, or VO_2, (muscular work capacity)[3] at rest in the morning and also four hours after exercise which would cancel out the elevation seen during exercise. This drop in VO_2 showed a progressive decline over the 3 week period in the exercise group as opposed to the non- exercise group where it remained relatively constant after an initial drop. The diet alone group did not show such declines after exercise, thereby, burning more calories during that time than the exercise group. This may explain why the additional energy used with exercise does not show up as added weight loss. Yet, we are bombarded by daily commercials and advertisements for weight loss through exercise and muscle

[2] The effect of exercise on RMR is discussed further in appendix III.

[3] Oxygen consumption (VO_2) is related directly to the amount of muscular work. Maximum oxygen uptake(or consumption), therefore, reflexes maximum work capacity. Many factors determine an individual's VO_2 such as age, gender, lean body, weight, genetic and most important the level of habitual exercise. Regular training for three month will increase the VO_2 by 30 to 40% where as three weeks of bed rest will cause a 20 to 25% decline in the VO_2. Therefore, the best overall measurement of the effect of training and of physical fitness is the maximum oxygen uptake (VO_2max). This is, also, equivalent to the state of cardiovascular fitness.

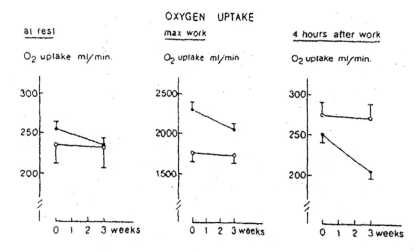

OXYGEN UPTAKE

at rest   max work   4 hours after work

Fig. 3.3 Oxygen uptake(metabolic rate) in the diet(500 kcal/day) alone group represented by open circles and diet plus exercise(55 minutes/3 times a week) represented by closed circles. The diet alone rate did not change over the 3 week period, however the diet plus exercise group showed a steady decline with a 4 hour rate significantly lower than diet alone. Krotkiewski, M., et al.(1981). The effect of a very-low-calorie diet with and without chronic exercise on thyroid and sex hormones, plasma proteins, oxygen uptake, insulin and c peptide concentrations in obese women. *Internat J of Obesity*, 5, 287-293. Reprinted by permission from Macmillian Publishers Ltd, copyright 1981.

building overlooking the truth. I believe that many of these programs do not take into account that the physiology is different during weight loss as compared to non-weight loss programs in which weight gain and increased food intake play major roles in increasing metabolism, both of which can not be part of a weight loss program. This leads to futile attempts of losing weight through the singular means of over- exercising resulting in failure and despair. This is not to say that exercise is unimportant and should be left out of a weight loss program. Figure 3.2 shows how lean body mass (mostly muscle) can be preserved during weight loss by exercise. We have seen how exercise is needed to overcome the reduction of the 24 hour TEE, non-resting energy component (Chapter 2).

How this is important in preventing weight regain (yo-yoing) as will be discussed in the next chapter. But exercise alone is not a means to lose weight nor does it accelerate weight loss when added to diet.

Chapter 4
Regain Rampage

Diary entry October 19th

I have loss 20# and I am at the same weight as my neighbor. But, how is it that she can eat more and exercise less and not gain?

Diary entry October 20th

Boy, if I miss one or two days of the exercise I notice immediately a one to two pound gain in my weight that week, even through I am eating the same things I did the first week that I lost weight.

This scenario points out the importance of exercise in maintaining weight. Therefore, the importance of exercise in a weight loss program isn't the fact that it reduces weight but it is a means of maintaining that new weight. A reduction in exercise is often the initiating act of weight gain.

There is justified pessimism regarding long term weight maintenance following weight loss programs. Successful weight maintenance is defined as a weight regain of less than 6.6 pounds in two years and a sustained reduction in waist circumference of at least 1.6 inches. In an average nutritional weight loss program two years after treatment only 2% maintained the weight loss of at least 20 pounds and in an average behavioral weight loss program only 2.6% of men and 28.9% of women had maintained 100% of their weight loss after four years.

There are many studies that show that physical inactivity after weight loss is predictive of greater weight regain. However, the one that best summarizes this and gives the best overall view of the importance of exercise, not in weight loss, but weight maintenance is seen in Figure 4.1. This study involved members of the Boston Police Department and metropolitan district commission who averaged 22% above ideal body weight. As can been seen on the left side of the graph the exercise and non-exercise groups loss weight roughly at the same rate with reduced-calorie diets during the first eight weeks. The weight loss that occurred during the reduced-calorie diet phase was almost completely wiped out for both groups who did not exercise during the follow-up period (47 and 8 at the top right corner). The most striking observation about this graph is found at the bottom right: following eight weeks of weight loss with diet alone three(3) of the non-exercise group began exercise and maintained their weight loss similar to those who exercised throughout both diet and follow up (36). In addition, unsupervised maintenance exercise during the follow-up phase (lines starting at 10, 52, 56 and 54) was shown to be as effective as supervised exercise (which occurred during the first 8 weeks) in this study when added to diet. The exercise consisted of three times a week at about 500 calories per session for a total of

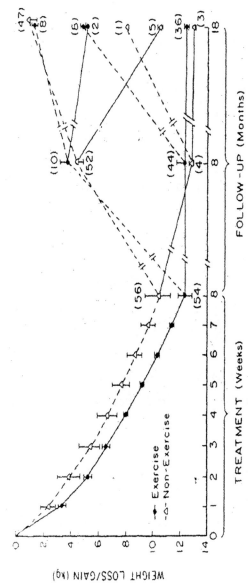

Fig. 4.1 Weight loss/gain over an 8 week treatment program and 18 month follow-up period. Treatment consisted of weekly diet instruction on either a 1000 kcal/day or 400-800 kcal/day diet, and the exercise group was required to exercise at 70-80% maximum heart rate for 30-60 minutes per day for three times a week under supervision. On the left side of the graph, exercise added little to weight loss, however, on the right side those that did not exercise gained back to their start weight over the 18 month follow-up, unlike those who exercised. Pavlou. Konstantin N., Krey,S., and William P. Steffee. (1989). Exercise as an adjunct to weight loss and maintenance in moderately obese subjects. *Am J Clin Nutr,* 49, 1115-23. Reproduced with permission from *The American Journal of Clinical Nutrition,* copyright, 1989.

1500 calories per week. This resulted in those who were successful in maintaining a reduced body weight. However, simple instruction without supervision during weight loss may not be adequate to reinforce activity changes in previously inactive subjects because only 5% of that group initiated exercise on their own.

As discussed in chapter 2, metabolic studies show a persistent decline in the metabolic rate that characterizes the reduced obese. Many studies show that the resting metabolic rate (RMR) decreases with diet induced weight loss by 15 to 30% below those at the same weight who have not loss (see figure 2.5). Although the drop in metabolism takes up to weeks to maximize, this reduced metabolic state can persist for up to 6 years, making for a predisposition back to obesity. Even though the post-obese individual can attain a body composition similar to lean individuals both in fat and lean content, the reduced metabolic state remains after weight loss. Furthermore, the reduced RMR can not be explained away as a loss of lean tissue (muscle) and this lowered metabolic state is not altered by exercise. As discussed in appendix III, there is no satisfactory scientific evidence that shows a prolonged increase in metabolic rate following intermittent exercise. Taken together the differences in the metabolic rates between the reduced-obese and always lean individuals are not related to changes in body composition or exercise, but seem to arise from differences in the efficiency of energy utilization in that the reduced individual requires less energy to function at the same weight as one who has never lost weight. The reason for this paradox still remains unexplained today.

These reduced-obese subjects, even when still overweight, require 15 to 30% fewer calories to maintain their new weight than subjects at that same weight who have not lost weight (control subjects). This appears to be a combination of not only a reduced metabolic rate, reduced work of movement at a lower body weight, reduced thermic effect of food (as fewer calories are eaten), but also, other energy regulatory homeostatic factors not fully understood at this time. Although this reduced metabolic state is important, other issues have their impact on regain. Over the past 14 years, I have observed a wide variability in the amount of weight regained from as little as 5 pounds to as much as 100 pounds. This would suggest that other exogenous factors contribute to weight regain other than the body attempting to re-establish its previous body composition and metabolic rate. Because of the wide variability of weight regain, these factors most likely involve not only poor adherence to physical activity, but re-emergence of bad eating habits with excess food intake having their impact on regaining.

The National Weight Control Registry (NWCR) collects data on individuals that have maintained a 30 pound weight loss for at least a year, but on average have maintained a 66 pound weight loss for 5.1 years. The key principles for *maintenance* of their weight loss were a combination of both increased physical activity and a low calorie diet. On average the diet closely resembles the moderate-fat, balanced nutrient *reduction* diet promoted by most health organizations for weight loss totaling around 1490 calories/day. This is considerably less than the 2500 calories per day eaten by the average US adult. Therefore, they are maintaining their weight on considerable lower calories than those who have not lost. Their physical activity is comparable to about 1 hour of moderate intensity, such as a brisk walk, per day. This is much higher than the Surgeon General's recommendations for the average adult of 30 minutes of moderate intensity activity at least 4 days/week. Among those individuals who regained their weight, there was a decrease in physical activity and dietary restraint, particularly loss of disinhibition (loss of control while eating, or binging). Those who have maintained their new weight for 2-5 years had a significant decrease in their risk of regaining. This underscores the importance of long term behavioral changes in diet and exercise that are needed to maintain weight loss.

Data from several studies indicate that the primary intervention for the prevention of weight gain in reduced obese individuals is associated with a threshold of 200 to 450 minutes of moderate intensity exercise per week (30 minutes to one hour a day). Less than that amount of exercise is accompanied by weight regain. In a follow up survey two years after a 500 kcal per day weight loss diet program, those who exercised (walking) more than 2000 kcal per week (walking 5 days a week) regained only 13% of their initial weight loss, whereas, those exercising at 1,200 kcal per week (walking 4 days a week) or 1000 kcal per week (2 days a week) had regained 72 and 75% of their weight loss, respectfully. Remember from chapter 2, the reduction in energy expenditure to 15-25% below that predicted for the slimmed weight as a result of a 10% decrease in body weight would be associated with a positive energy balance of about 375 kcal/day. This intensity of exercise at a minimum ranges from as little as 60 to 75% maximum heart rate for 45 minutes per day for five days a week targeting an energy equivalent of 400 calories per session or 2000 calories per week, to as much as one to 1.3 hours a day at the same intensity level aiming for 2500 to 3000 calories per week. This intensity corresponds to the greatest fat utilization occurring at 55 to 72% of the aerobic capacity.[1] See figure 4.2. Less fat burning occurs at higher or lower rates of exercise.

[1]Aerobic capacity (or work capacity) is the maximal capability to transport and utilize oxygen during movement without the buildup of lactate (lactic acid). The American College of Sports Medicine recommends exercising at 60-90% maximum heart rate for 30-60 minutes on 3.5 days a week for aerobic fitness. Maximal heart rate may be predicted by subtracting age from 220. Aerobic exercises are those that use large muscle groups and are continuous and rhythmic, such as walking.

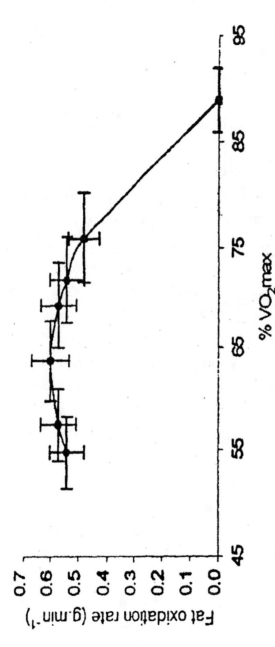

Fig. 4.2 Fat oxidation (burning or utilitization) versus exercise intensity expressed as percentage of VO$_{2max}$(maximum uptake of oxygen or work capacity). The greatest amount of fat burning occurs at 55%-72% of maximum exercise effort. Achten, Juul, Gleeson, Michael, and Jeukendrup, Asker. (2002). Determination of the exercise intensity that elicits maximal fat oxidation. *Med Sci Sports Exer*, 34(1), 92-97. Permission granted Lippincott, Williams, and Wilkins copyright, 2002.

A study of overweight women on reducing diets showed that shorts bouts of exercise (a ten minute bout four times a day) versus a single 40 minute bout/day resulted in a significantly greater number of days on which exercise was done and the number of times it was completed than the single, long bout. This would suggest that at short bouts of exercise may improve exercise adherence and as a result improve weight maintenance. By increasing activity to a level of brisk walking (4mph) 16 to 20 miles per week (2,000 kcal per week) or more than 200 minutes per week spread over at least 5 days a week (40 minutes/day), the reduced-obese individual can improve the chance for long term success. See figure 4.3. Current recommendations by the Surgeon General for 30 minutes a day, 4 days a week would result in less than 150 minutes/week, which would correspond to the top curve in figure 4.3 and result in weight gain. Although more time most be put into exercise than those who have never been overweight, a Herculean effort is not required. Nonetheless, the intensity of the exercise is as important as the duration as depicted figure 4.4. After recent weight loss to ideal body weight, moderate activity (walking at 3.3 mph for 50 minutes/day/7 days a week) was no different from sedentary activity (walking at 3.3 mph for 40 minutes/day/7 days a week) as both resulted in a gradual weight gain over the year. However, increasing the intensity to an active level of walking at 3.3 mph for 80 minutes/day or 4 mph for 36 minutes/day/7 days a week resulted in no weight gain. This active level of activity results in a 70-80% maximal heart rate (effort), which would permit an individual to talk while exercising continuously for 20-60 minutes improving fitness and health without exacerbating joint pain even for those with arthritic joints. For most the difficulty of a commitment is not the intensity of the exercise but finding the time.

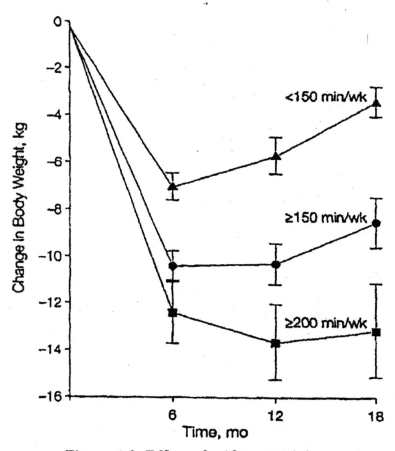

Figure 4.3 Effect of self-reported time spent exercising following a 6 month weight loss period of 148 sedentary, overweight women. Those that reported 200 or more minutes per week of exercise tended not to regain. Jakicic, JM, Winters,C, Lang, W, and Wing, RR. (1999), Effects of intermittent exercise and use of home equipment on adherence, weight loss, and fitness in overweight women: a randomized trial. *JAMA*,282(16), 1554-1560. With permission of the AMA, copyright 1999.

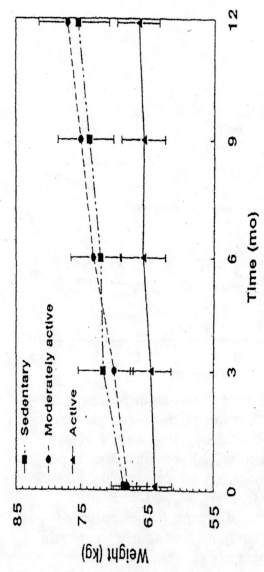

Fig.4.4 Average body weights in three groups of previously obese women in the year after completion of weight loss. Increases in weight were significantly less in active women. Schoeller, Dale A., Shay, Kathyjo, and Kushner, Robert F. (1997). How much physical activity is needed to minimize weight gain in previously obese women? *Am J Clin Nutr*, 66, 551–6. Permission granted by the American Society for Nutrition, copyright 1997.

In light of all these findings, maintenance of weight loss requires a lifetime of commitment because of the potentially dangerous effect of the high rates of recidivism (weight loss/gain cycles).[2] Furthermore, this commitment requires a higher standard of effort in maintaining a greater vigilance to a lower calorie diet and an elevated level of habitual exercise as compared to others who have not reduced. A weight loss commitment does not stop after achieving the desired weight, but in many ways becomes tougher to maintain. Whereas weight loss can occur simply by a reduced diet, maintenance of weight loss requires both a daily regulation of diet and exercise. The reduced diet needs to average 1000 calories less than others at the same weight who have not been obese, and must be based on adherence to behavioral changes in coping with social and personal stressors. A daily exercise program must be maintained that is higher than the 1995 joint recommendation of the Centers for Disease Control and the American College of Sports Medicine of 30 minutes/day of moderate activity to promote health and reduce disease. The exercise program after weight loss, also, exceeds the 30 minutes/ day of moderate-intensity activity or 15 minutes/day of vigorous activity recommended by the Surgeon General for preservation of health. Therefore, obesity should be thought of as a chronic disease much in the same way as we consider hypertension: never cured, but controlled. Continued vigilance is required to prevent weight regain.

[2]The fluctuation of weight seems to carry a higher risk of mortality than stable obesity. See chapter 9.

Chapter 5
Homeostasis Harmony

Diary entry December 7th

I afraid that if I lose weight too fast that I will lose so much muscle that when I regain I will be too weak to try to lose again. I get weak and dizzy at times, so I eat to bring up my blood sugar. After all, the brain needs sugar to work.

This scenario discusses the series of metabolic and hormonal changes that occur as body transitions from the fed state to a brief fasting period and then into prolonged calorie restriction. Although this book is intended for the general population it is also intended for the medical profession. To those without medical expertise this chapter may be laborious but at the same time intriguing.

Weight loss involves the transition from obtaining the majority of energy from food eaten to primarily utilizing the energy stored in the body. The body's stored energy is distributed into three separate compartments: glycogen, protein, fat. Fat constitutes 85% of the stored energy and since it requires very little water it has the most energy (calories) per gram thereby maximizing storage efficiency. Fat stores are considered relatively inert and need time to get up and running, and then, only after the right signals are received. Unlike fat, glycogen is in constant flux, being depleted during sleep or exercise only to be replenished by the next meal. It is a quick and ready source of energy. However, it is in very limited supply being only 2.5% of the body's total stored energy. As one would imagine this source is quickly used up. To bridge the time from glycogen depletion (24 hours) up to ten days when fat begins to mobilize to provide the majority of the body's energy needs, there is a shift from using glycogen to breaking down and reconstructing proteins of the body to provide amino acids to be turned into glucose for supplying the body's energy needs (gluconeogensis).[1] Because of the functional and structural importance of protein to support life there is a need to limit its breakdown. Therefore, there is a lifesaving downshift in the rate of protein breakdown at two to ten days following the onset of weight loss to conserve protein by mobilizing fat stores (lipolysis/ketogenesis) to provide the majority of the body's energy needs. This *critical event* in the adaptation sequence during weight loss allows survival to be extended from 60 days to over 260 days provided that adequate fluid and electrolytes are provided. This sequence of metabolic events occurring with weight loss from decrease food intake (as a result of dieting or fasting) occurs in a predictable and reproducible pattern as depicted in figure 5.1

[1]Skeletal muscle can not release glucose directly from its stored glycogen, however, it gets around this by releasing lactate and amino acids such as alanine, which can be converted to glucose in the liver.

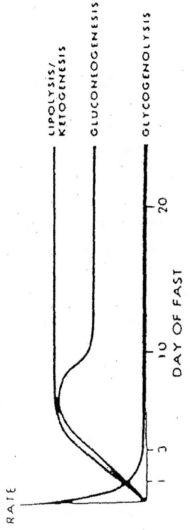

Fig. 5.1 Changes in rates of glycogenolysis, gluconeogenesis, lipolysis and ketogenesis that are required to maintain glucose homeostasis from brief to prolonged fasting. Kerndt,PR, Naughton,JL, Driscoll,CE, and Loxterkamp,DA. (1982). Fasting: the history, pathophysiology and complications. *West J Med*, 137, 379-399. Reproduced with permission from the BMJ Publishing Group, copyright 1982.

Despite the small limited stores of carbohydrate (glucose) in glycogen, a continuous supply of glucose is essential for survival, even during the time in which fat is being broken down as the primary energy source as ketones and fatty acids. Although reliance of the brain on glucose diminishes (50 to 68% reduction) with weight loss, there is still a residual glucose requirement by the brain. Furthermore, other tissues such as the cells of the bone marrow, peripheral nerves, red and white corpuscles and the kidney have an obligate requirement for glucose for anaerobic metabolism (breakdown of glucose to lactate and pyruvate).[2] Early in weight loss muscle's glycogen is broken down to provide energy as lactate which is released into the blood and restructured back into glucose by the liver and kidney. This Cori cycle does not provide an increase in glucose or energy since the lactate was originally derived from glucose, and the energy used to re-sensitize the glucose off sets that derived from its breakdown. However, there are advantages provided by this cycle. First, the energy for hepatic (liver) glucose synthesis is from fatty acid breakdown so that this new glucose molecule can now be utilized for energy having used fat as its source for resynthesis.[3] Secondly, this recycling decreases the need for protein derived glucose, sparing protein breakdown.

After most of the glycogen stores are depleted by the first 24 hours of weight loss, protein is broken down to provide amino acids for reconstructing into glucose for energy. Alanine, which constitutes 7 to 10% of skeletal muscle accounts for 30 to 40% of all the amino acids released into the blood stream from muscles during

[2]These cells lack mitochondria. These small organelles (organ within an organ) are capable of taking the anaerobic byproducts of the breakdown of glucose to pyruvate to further extract energy with the release of CO_2 and water. The mitochondria is the place where aerobic metabolism occurs.
[3]Mammals lack enzymes to change fatty acid back to glucose directly.

this time. It appears that the majority (60 to 70%) of the alanine coming from muscle is derived from pyruvate (the end product of the breakdown of glucose) joining with nitrogen donated by a group of branched amino acids. Subsequently, this alanine is released into the blood and resynthesized into glucose by the liver.[4] This glucose-alanine cycle provides two different control points for the inhibition of gluconeogensis. With refeeding blood glucose levels increase with a resultant increase in insulin, which reduces gluconeogensis by inhibiting liver uptake of alanine. With continued weight loss there is an increase in ketones from fat breakdown that slows gluconeogensis by decreasing the degradation of branched amino acids, which supply the nitrogen to form alanine. Either way, whether the individual is fed or continues to restrict intake, there is a point in time that gluconeogenesis is diminished.

Although early on the liver is the primary site of producing new glucose, the kidney gradually assumes almost half the total glucose production as weight loss continues. The kidney, however, prefers to extract glucose from glutamine instead of alanine with the nitrogen containing byproduct of ammonia instead of urea (as with the alanine cycle).[5] See Figure 5.2. This change has several adaptative advantages. First, the positively charged ammonia produced can neutralize the negatively charged ketones to prevent their dangerous build up in the blood in place of sodium (which

[4]During the early phase of weight loss the liver is the sole source of blood glucose. In as much as liver glycogen stores are depleted within the first three days of weight loss. This glucose production relies heavily on lactate and amino acid substrates to keep pace with the rapid rate of glucose utilization by the brain during this time.
[5] Muscle/amino acids contain nitrogen, therefore, there would be a build up of nitrogen left over after breaking down glutamine or alanine, unless this excess nitrogen is eliminated. Nitrogen is excreted from the body in the form of urea or ammonia in the urine and stool, so measuring their loss is a measure of muscle/protein loss.

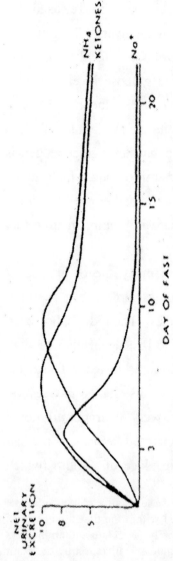

Fig. 5.2 The urinary excretion of sodium(Na⁺), ketones and ammonium(NH₄) during fasting. Sodium losses decrease as ammonium becomes available as a cation(positively charged molecule) to be excreted with ketones(negatively charged). Ketone losses decrease with increased renal reabsorption; this is accompanied by a decreased ammonium excretion. Kerndt,PR, Naughton,JL, Driscoll,CE, and Loxterkamp,DA.(1982).Fasting: the history, pathophysiology and complications. West J Med, 137,379-399. Reproduced with from the BMJ Publishing Group, copyright 1982.

is, also, positively charged) thereby significantly reducing the accelerated loss of sodium and water associated with the early phase of weight loss. Secondly, unlike urea, ammonia, can be reabsorbed,(seen as a reduction in its excretion with prolonged fasting) reducing the nitrogen loss seen with hepatic derived urea, thereby, reducing the breakdown of protein to supply this nitrogen.

During this later phase of weight loss which is directed at protein conservation now, hepatic gluconeogensis is reduced to 40 to 50 grams per day compared. Although the kidney is now contributing an additional 40 grams per day of glucose, the total availability of glucose is far less than required at the start of weight loss. In the fed state the human body requires 150 to 250 grams of glucose per day with the brain consuming 125 to 150 grams per day while resting muscle and obligate cells consume the rest. This problem is solved by the brain shifting its energy requirements to ketones which as weight loss continues, will account for 50 to 60% of its needs[6]. Yet, blood glucose levels remain normal during all this time. With the decrease in brain utilization of blood glucose there has to be a decrease in the production of new glucose and this seems to be due primarily to the reduction of hepatic glucose production (gluconeogensis) induced by the fall in alanine, brought on by the inhibition of branched amino acid transfer of nitrogen to alanine by the elevated ketones. See Figure 5.4.

There are other regulators of this cascade of metabolic changes induced by weight loss. Two of these are insulin and glucagon which are hormones produced by the pancreas. The early phase of weight

---

[6]Also, during a fast of more than 24 hours, muscle and fatty tissues utilization of glucose virtually crease. Muscle in early fasting relies on ketones for energy, but with prolonged fasting muscle metabolism shifts from ketones to fatty acids.

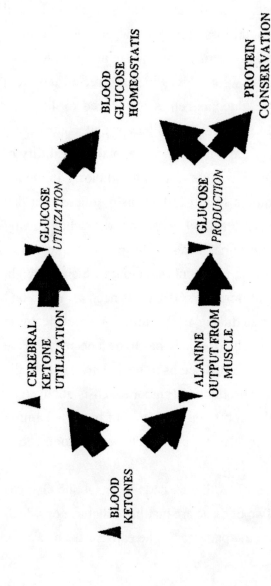

Fig. 5.4 The late metabolic adaptation of starvation. Ketones replace glucose as the main substrate for the brain (decreased glucose utilization) and signal a reduction of alanine from muscle (decreased glucose production) causing a reduction of protein breakdown. Both of these changes produce a normalization of blood glucose. Saudek,Christopher D. and Felig, Philip. (1976). The metabolic events of starvation. *Am J Med*, 60, 117-126. Reprinted with permission from Elsevier, copyright 1976.

loss induces a fall in insulin and a rise in glucagon levels in the blood.[7] These changes facilitate an outpouring of amino acids and fatty acids into the blood stream. Low insulin promotes peripheral fat/protein breakdown, whereas, glucagon stimulates the release of glycogen from the liver and, also, stimulates uptake of the alanine for gluconeogensis. These changes help to maintain the blood glucose level at near normal during this time.

However, this sequence of events can be disrupted by ingestion of as little as 50 to 100 grams per day of carbohydrate. At this amount the digested carbohydrates will appreciably raise the blood glucose and with that insulin levels will increase thereby reducing fat breakdown to ketones (ketosis). But, an intake of one gram of protein per 2.2 pounds (1kg) of body weight (which is 114 grams for a 250 pound person) does not inhibit ketosis and results only in a modest elevation of insulin[8]. This provides an explanation for the success of weight loss diets that include variable amounts of protein but little or no carbohydrates Their primary goal is to keep insulin levels low to promote the breakdown of fat.

In summary, the human metabolic response to diet-induced weight loss involves changes in hormones and utilization of different energy stores. The initial and late phases are significantly different as the body shifts from maintaining blood glucose at all costs to minimizing the rate of protein breakdown. Whereas, the initial phase is characterized by the need to maintain high levels of glucose production for the brain by liver utilization of protein breakdown (gluconeogensis) with nitrogen loss as urea, the late phase is characterized by the decreased need for glucose with increasing reliance on ketones by the brain, and the kidney assuming a more important role in gluconeogensis with

---

[7] Please, refer to chapter 8 for more details about insulin and glucagon.
[8] Please, refer to figure 6.3 in chapter 6 which shows that increase intake of protein preserves body protein without inhibiting ketosis.

ammonia byproducts which result in less nitrogen loss from protein. With weight loss there is a shift from a predominantly glucose based energy source from glycogen and protein to one that relays primarily on ketones and fatty acids from fat. Primary regulators of this initial response are the reduction in plasma insulin and increase in glucagon. For millions of years this biphasic response has allowed humans to adapt to starvation for several months while maintaining a sufficient level of energy to meet the body's needs and physical activity.

Chapter 6
Protein Puzzle

Diary entry October 10th

I worry that if I lose weight I will lose muscle. But, if I work out I will change fat to muscle and stop losing. After all, muscle weighs more than fat.

In discussing the loss of protein (muscle or lean body mass) during weight loss one has to remember that all proteins of the body serve a structural or metabolic function. Therefore, bodily functions can be impaired if proteins are broken down for energy without being replaced. The concept of lethal weight loss from starvation is based on how much protein can be lost before death. In 1921 it was Krieger who postulated that the lethal weight loss in humans was about 40% during acute and 50% during semi-starvation. However, currently gastric bypass patients may lose as much as 35% of body weight over a period of 7 to 12 months with almost all mortality related only to the surgical procedure or peri-operative (occurring around the time of the surgery) complications and not related to the weight loss. Even with this happening so blatantly, many in the field of health care stick to the dogma of successful weight loss as a safe one to two pound per week aiming for a 10% total weight reduction. Old myths die hard.

Autopsy findings in humans dying from starvation show a loss of 25 to 50% lean tissue from organs with almost complete loss of fat at the time of death. So if the loss of protein during starvation was the same for lean individuals as for obese individuals then obese individuals would die with most of their fat stores in place and should not be able to survive much longer than their lean companions. However there is plenty of evidence that although lean human beings die between 57 to 73 days from starvation losing about 40% of their body weight, there are several reports of obese individuals who have starved for more than 100 days and survived.

Although obese people have more protein (fat free mass) than lean individuals this does not explain the prolonged survival time during starvation. Breakdown of protein correlates with the loss of nitrogen in urine. So the higher the breakdown of protein in the body, the higher the levels of nitrogen in urine. During weight loss obese individuals have lower nitrogen excretion in urine than lean individuals. This difference becomes apparent only after the first week of starvation with significant differences developing by the third week. See Figure 6.1. Two major observations can be made from this graph. First, the loss of nitrogen (breakdown of protein) in reducing obese individuals is three to four times lower than that of lean individuals after the first three weeks of starvation. Second, the values in lean people do not appear to decline with time as they do with the obese. Therefore, the obese lose an increasingly smaller proportion of lean tissue as weight reduction continues than lean individuals. In addition, those individuals with lowest BMI (20)

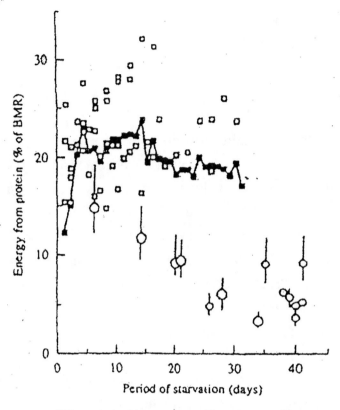

Fig. 6.1 The contribution of energy
from protein to basal metabolic
rate(BMR) during starvation in
lean(squares) and obese(circles)
subjects. Elia, M. (2000). Hunger
disease. *Clin Nutr*, 19(6), 379-386.
Reprinted with permission from
Elsevier, copyright 2000.

and smallest amount of initial body fat may derive five times more of the basal (resting) energy expenditure from protein breakdown than obese individuals with more fat associated with a BMI of 40 or more. Furthermore, the ratio of lean-tissue loss to total body weight is *inversely* related to the initial fat mass during reduced food intake (*an inverse relationship is defined as one factor goes down, in this case--lean-tissue loss, the other factor goes up, in this case--initial fat mass is higher*). Therefore, the obese lose less lean-tissue during weight loss than lean individuals on the same reduction diet. Results from 40 post gastric bypass patients are shown in Figure 6.2. Despite continuing fat loss, lean body mass which was initially lost in the first three months can be restored while weight loss continues. This restoration is due in some part to the increase in protein intake after three months, but restoration of lean-tissue with simultaneous fat loss is not seen in lean individuals undergoing weight loss. The metabolic processes that recognize and allow for these different responses between lean and obese individuals are not understood and remain to be explained.

Not only does the amount of fat that an individual carries produce differences in protein loss during dieting, but the macronutrient (type of food e.g. carbs) can cause changes in the amount of fat/protein loss. As shown in Figure 6.3 small amounts of protein, (for instance 40gm) can prevent loss of nitrogen in urine as it occurs in starvation while the breakdown of fat (represented as ketones in urine, ketonuria) continues. Higher amounts of protein (80grams), however, diminish the breakdown of fat which results in a drop in ketonuria. The addition of only 40 grams of carbohydrates (unlike 40 grams of protein) will not prevent nitrogen loss (loss of muscle/protein) in urine but will reduce ketonuria (ketones loss in urine). See figure 6.4. Also, shown in figure 6.4 is that dietary fat supplementation does

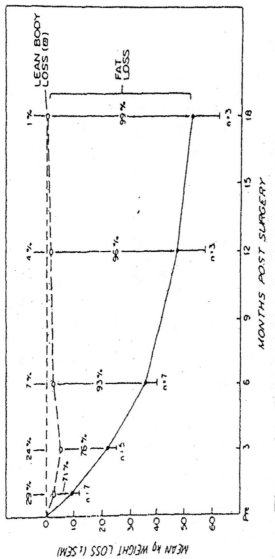

Figure 6.2 Composition of weight loss following gastric bypass. Note continued fat loss with preservation of lean tissue. Bothe, Albert, Bistrian,BR, Greenberg,I,and Blackburn,GL. (1979). Energy regulation in morbid obesity by multicisplinary theraphy. *Surg Clin N Am*, 59(6), 1017-1031.Reprinted with permission from Elsevier,© 1979.

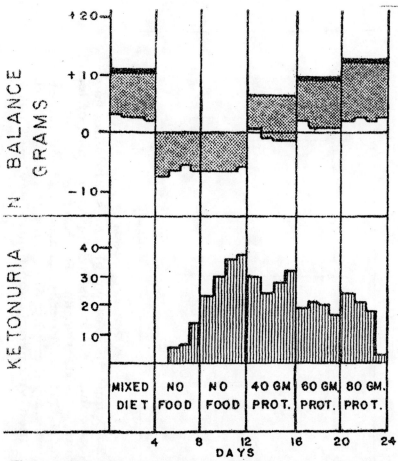

Figure 6.3 The effect on nitrogen(N) balance during starvation with increasing amounts of protein intake is represented by the upper graph. The effect on ketonuria (ketones in the urine) in arbitrary units is shown in the lower graph during the same time. At 40 grams/day of protein intake, one obtains a positive affect on nitrogen balance (preservation of body protein) without significantly suppressing ketonuria(fat breakdown by-product). Bollinger,RE,et al. (1966). Metabolic balance of obese subjects during fasting. *Arch Intern Med*, 118,3-8. With permission by the AMA, © 1966.

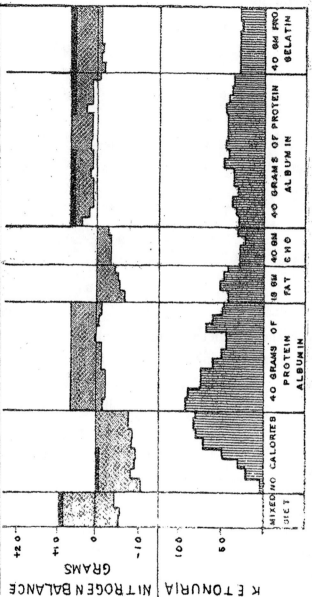

Figure 6.4 Nitrogen balance (top graph) and ketonuria (bottom graph) during various additions of protein, fat, and carbohydrate(CHO) to a starvation diet. The mixed diet period is equal to 4 days and the other time periods are proportionate on the graph (about 4 days for the small boxes and 12 days for the larger boxes). Positive nitrogen balance (preservation of body protein) is seen with addition of protein without loss of ketonuria (breakdown by-products of fat loss), whereas fat and CHO do not conserve nitrogen. Bollinger, RE, et al. (1966). Metabolic balance of obese subjects during fasting. *Arch Intern Med*, 118,3-8. With permission of the AMA,© 1966.

not spare nitrogen loss but has less effect on reducing fat breakdown as do carbohydrates.

The quantity and source of protein catabolism (process of breaking down) during weight loss is of major importance. Obese individuals have a higher oxygen uptake (VO_2max) or work capacity at rest and at sub-maximal work loads when compared to normal weight individuals, which results most likely from the greater muscle mass required by obese individuals to carry the extra weight. It is thought that it may contribute to an "extra tissue protein" pool that is broken down in place of muscle during weight loss. The exact nature of this non-muscle protein pool is not known, but several studies have strongly suggested its existence.

To test if muscle/strength loss occurs with the protein loss during weight reduction, male, Boston police volunteers who where free of known serious medical disorders and 20% or more over ideal body weight were placed in a study. These police officers were placed on an 800 kcal per day diet and either rested or exercised on a treadmill from 70 to 85% of maximum heart rate three times a week. This exercise program has been found to be adequate to produce a cardiovascular fitness effect (cardiovascular training) as measured by VO_2. These findings are shown in figure 6.5. These graphs show that a progressive (starting at 70% and working up to 85% maximum heart rate) exercise program added to a low calorie, reducing diet can result in (1) preservation of existing lean body tissue; (2) increase fat loss; (3) increase VO_2 max (or cardiovascular fitness); and (4) increase in strength during weight loss. The increase in strength without an increase in total body weight as seen in this study apparently occurs as a result of an exercise-induced capacity to simultaneously recruit greater numbers of muscle fibers as occurs with training, or, a redistribution of lean body mass occurs, increasing

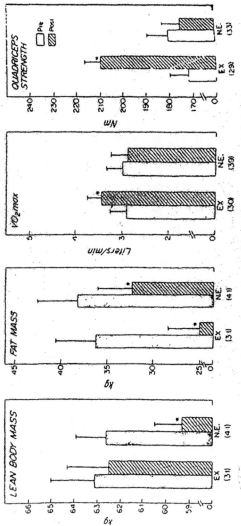

Fig. 6.5 Changes in lean body mass, fat mass, VO₂max, and quadriceps strength during an 800 kcal/day diet over 8 weeks. The 72 obese subjects were divided into exercise(EX) and non-exercise(NE) groups. Exercise consisted of a walk/jog at 70-85% maximum heart rate. The number of subjects studied are in parenthesis and the small stars represent a significant change from the start(Pre) to the end(Post) of testing. Although there were significant gains in VO₂max and Quads strength in the EX group, there was no significant determent in these two factors in those who did not exercise(NE). Also, there was no significant difference in total weight loss between the two groups even though there was a difference in changes in lean body mass and fat mass. Pavlou, Konstantin N, Steffee, WP,Herman,RH, and Burrows,BA. (1985). Effects of dieting and exercise on lean body mass, oxygen uptake, and strength. *Med Sci Sporte Exerc*, 17(4), 466-471. Reprinted with permission by Lippincott, Williams, and Wilkins, copyright 1985.

the mass of the stressed muscle groups at the expense of an "extra protein tissue" pool.

In a comparative study of resistant weight training vs. non-weight training, obese females were placed on 1,000 kcal per day deficient diet. As expected from other studies, there was no significant difference in weight loss between diet only vs. diet plus exercise (see chapter 3). However, resistance exercise during a weight loss diet produced similar gain in lean tissue as compared to those not on a diet. In the same study the rate of strength gain or magnitude of upper arm area increase was the same as compared to those with exercise without caloric restriction. Although the diet only group did lose lean body weight it did not correspond to decrease strength or radiographic muscle area. One would, therefore, suspect that there are moderate lean tissue losses throughout the body and these losses are for the most part from non-muscle protein pool, otherwise, one would not have seen the gains in strength if the lean tissue weight loss came from muscle.

Resting metabolic rate (RMR) decreases with weight loss and is not increased with exercise training despite a substantial training induced increase in physical fitness (VO_2max) unlike what happens in those not losing weight. In a study done at Emory University, obese women on an 800 kcal per day diet and walking 5.6 kilometers every three days experienced a continued decline in RMR as did non-exercising dieters, even though the exercisers had lost less lean body weight (or fat free mass, FFM).[1] The total RMR decline was 19% in exercisers and 17.3% in non-exercisers at the end of the 6 week diet. Therefore, the decline in RMR cannot be attenuated by

---

[1] Lean body weight (FFM, Fat Free Mass) is considered metabolically active as opposed to fat, which is considered inactive. Although exercise preserves FFM, it does not preserve the RMR (Resting Metabolic Rate). For more on RMR see chapter 2 and appendix III.

exercise and can not be explained solely by the loss of FFM (or lean protein mass).

Obese women on a weight reducing 544 kcal per day diet for four weeks showed a transitory decrease in muscle strength (knee extension), but stabilized after the first two weeks with no further decrease in muscle strength. However, there was improvement in the muscle endurance during the next two weeks with no further improvement after another two weeks. It has been seen that in obese patients who have lost at least 20% of their body mass following vertical banded gastroplasty, there was significant improvement in respiratory muscle endurance after six months. These findings differ from patients with anorexia nervosa (who go form normal weight to underweight) in whom the muscles not only generate less power but tire easily and relax slowly.

These observations suggest that weight loss is different in obese individuals as compared to lean. Not only do obese individuals have a slower turn over in protein but the rate at which protein is lost during weight reduction is less.[2] The metabolic process that underlie these differences are not known at this time. The muscle wasting that occurs in lean individuals during weight loss must not be inferred for reducing obese individuals. In fact the protein loss in reducing-obese individuals, who exercise, is not associated with loss of strength and actual gains in strength and endurance can occur. Furthermore, lean tissue loss during weight reduction in the obese can be reduced by adding the optimal amount of protein to the diet and an exercise program of mild-to moderate intensity.

---

[2]There is no escape from the fact that significant weight loss in humans is almost always accompanied by a loss of lean body mass (LBM) as well as fat. The only exception in the animal world is the hibernating bear. During winter sleep the bear loses only fat (up to 13% of initial weight). However, when the bear is fasted during the summer, it loses LBM as well as fat.

Chapter 7
Genetic Gripe

Diary entry January 26th

I was not fat until I got pregnant. Having babies must reduce a woman's metabolism causing fat.

Diary entry January 27th

I talked to my sister today. She states that the reason why I cannot lose weight is because of genetics. Indeed everyone in the family is fat except for Aunt Hattie who came over from the "old country", who is long gone now.

Information regarding whether obesity is inherited or not comes from two major sources: DNA and population studies. For many years obesity in rodents has been known to be caused by a number of single gene deletions or mutations that cause both hyperphagia (increased appetite) and diminished energy expenditure, suggesting a link between these two parameters of energy homeostasis.

Identification of the *ob* gene mutation in genetic obese mice (*ob/ob*) represented a major breakthrough in the field of obesity genetics. It was found that the product of the *ob* gene is a peptide produced by adipose cells called leptin. The mutation in the *ob/ob* mice resulted in a leptin deficiency that led to obesity. It appears that leptin is secreted by the adipose cells and acts primarily on the hypothalamus (lower part of the brain) to decrease food intake and increase energy expenditure. Both of these defects were reversed by treatment with leptin and therefore lead to a search for a *candidate gene* in humans.[1] The *ob* gene is found to be present in humans and expressed in fat. This began an explosion in the study for a genetic basis to obesity. However, the genetic deficency of leptin is a very rare cause of human obesity. In fact most obese humans have elevated levels of leptin representing a leptin resistant state. However, a number of complex human syndromes with well defined inheritance are associated with obesity. One of these is the Prader-Willi syndrome which is a congenital disorder characterized by obesity, mental retardation, and hypogonadism (lack of sexual maturity). This obese condition is due to a very small deletion or mutation of chromosome 15. Studies of Mexican-Americans and Pima Indians have revealed strong positional candidate genes for obesity on chromosomes 2 and 8.

At a population level the genetic component of obesity is expressed in terms of heritability. This refers to the proportion of the total variation in a characteristic which is attributable to genetic factors. But, differences in genetic susceptibility within a population may actually determine which individuals are more likely to become obese when exposed to certain changes in their environment. This would imply that environmental factors (availability of food, machinery to

---

[1]Candidate genes are genes identified on the basis of the effects in animal studies with suspected physiological involvement in a particular disorder in humans.

replace hard labor, etc.) would play the dominate role in determining which trait was allowed to be expressed. Therefore, even if a person had the gene for obesity, that person could be lean unless exposed to factors that would promote obesity such as inactivity or over-eating. The following observations have been made in an attempt to determine what factors have a role in the etiology of obesity.

A study of adoptees in Denmark found that 80% of off spring of two obese parents become obese as compared to 14% of the offspring of two parents of normal weight. No relationship was found between the adoptee and adoptive parents whether the adoptive parents were obese or not, suggesting that the childhood family environment had little or no effect. However, in a study done in Puget Sound, Washington, parental obesity more than doubled the risk of adult obesity among both obese and non-obese children before the age of six years, but was less an influence after the age of 10 years. Among *non-obese* one and two year olds, those with at least one obese parent had a greater chance of being obese as adults (28%) than those without an obese parent (10%). If the 1-2 years olds were *obese*, the chance of becoming an obese adult rose from 8% if neither parent was obese to 40% if at least one parent was obese. Among *obese* 3 to 5 year olds, the chance of adult obesity increased from 24% if neither parent was obese to 62% if at least one parent was obese. Before the age of 3 years the parents' obesity status was the primary predictor of that child being an obese adult; between the ages of 3 to 9 years, the child's and parents' obesity status were both important predictors; but, at older ages the child's obesity status alone became more important.[2] This would suggest environmental factors become

[2] Obese children under the age of 3 years should not be labeled as being at risk for later obesity if the parents are not obese. In contrast, any 1to 2 year old who has an obese parent, especially both, is at risk of later obesity. There is no significant difference in risk due to the sex of the child.

more influential after the age of 10 years in the expression of obesity, in genetically susceptible children.

The Quebec family study is shown in the schematic pie summary (figure 7.1). Although the genetic contribution was from 5 to 30% (the greater contribution for an internal, or deep, fat pattern of distribution as opposed to superficial or fat just beneath the skin), the transmissible component from generation to generation was primarily cultural (non-genetic) and that the non-transmissible influences (environmental) usually had more important effect than the genetic components. In the above mentioned Danish adoptee study the estimate of heritability of BMI was 34% suggesting that the remaining variation of BMI was mostly due to non-shared environmental effects. These studies closely agree, therefore, that there appears to be a 30% genetic influence on obesity, but, an overwhelming 60% impact by environmental factors

It would appear that environmental factors play a critical role in the development in obesity by unmasking genetic or metabolic susceptibilities. When a dramatic change in the diet and lifestyle occurred in the Naura of Micronesia and the Polynesians of Western Somalia, the prevalence of obesity shot up to over 60%. Migrations, where populations with a common genetic heritage now live under different environments, can cause a significant unmasking of genetic/metabolic susceptibilities to obesity.[3] The Pima Indians living in the U.S.A. average 25 kilograms heavier than those living in Mexico.

---

[3] The "thrifty" genotype hypothesis proposes that genes which enhance carriers to more easily assimilate food as fat thereby conferring a survival benefit in their original habitat where food is scarce, would predispose those to obesity when the population enters an environment where food is abundant

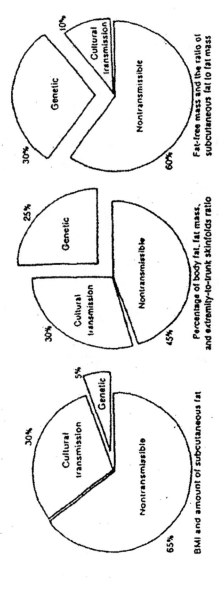

Fig. 7.1 The major affectors of human variation in body composition and fat distribution obtained from 1698 members of 409 families of French descent. There appears to be a very small contribution of biological inheritance to the body mass index and the amount of subcutaneous fat (skin folds), but a larger contribution to the fat mass, fat-free mass, and fat distribution. Bouchard, Claude, et al. (1988). Inheritance of the amount and distribution of human body fat. *International J of Obesity*, 12, 205-215. Reprinted by permission from Macmillian Publishers Ltd, copyright 1988.

Migrant Africans living in the Caribbean or U.S.A. show a significant increase in the prevalence of obesity in comparison to their native countries of Nigeria or Cameroon. With the increase in obesity, adverse health consequences emerge such as hypertension, which ranges from only about 15% in those living in Africa to over 30% among those in the United States.

Environmental influences have an effect through increasing energy intake or decreasing energy expenditure to cause obesity. Some studies have shown that as the proportion of dietary fat increases there is a significant increase in the prevalence of obesity in both men and women. Cross cultural studies of physical activity and BMI have shown a significant increased risk of overweight in those less active with an increased likelihood of becoming obese. In a large Finish study those reporting physical exercise three or more times per week had on average lost weight since a preceding survey five years earlier. Those with little physical activity, however, had gained weight and had twice the risk of gaining in excess of 5kg than the physically active subjects.

Depending on the predominant source of energy that is being utilized the ratio of carbon dioxide production to consumption of oxygen (RQ) will vary. The RQ decreases when fat is the predominant source of metabolism as in dieting or starvation and increases when the contribution of carbohydrate increases as occurs with overfeeding. There is evidence that the RQ for an individual is under genetic influence. When controlling for food preferences, twin studies and cross cultural population studies have suggested a genetic heritability of RQ of 20 to 45%.[4] Those individuals with a high RQ were found to be more likely to gain weight than those with a low RQ (reflecting

---

[4]This is similar to the 30% heritability seen in the previous discussed Danish adoptee and Quebec family studies.

a high utilization of fat). These studies suggest that there may be a heritable influence on the ability to utilize carbohydrates over fat as the primary fuel for energy that would predispose certain individuals to gain weight when exposed to an environment of high fat intake and low physical activity. These individuals would be expected to have a high prevalence of obesity, whether they migrated to, or adopted, an environment high in fatty food availability.

In experiments where lean and obese adults were overfed the same amount, no difference was observed in the rate of weight gain. Furthermore, in women who became obese during or shortly after pregnancy, no reduction in resting metabolic rate as a result of pregnancy was found that would cause their obesity. Therefore, there appears to be no specific, genetic defect in metabolism that would predispose a diverse population of adults to obesity or be activated as a result of pregnancy.

The combined evidence of these genetic studies suggests that obesity is a disorder of multiple genes that are susceptible to environmental influences, but do not alter the resting metabolism. The occurrence of these genes increases the risk of developing obesity, but are not essential by themselves to cause the development of obesity. This means that environmental factors play a decisive role in unmasking latent genetic tendencies to develop obesity by means as yet unknown. Therefore, the differences in genetic susceptibility determines which individuals are more likely to become obese in a given set of environmental circumstances.

Chapter 8
Hormones Hyped

Diary entry November 15th

I cannot seem to lose weight. Ruth thinks I should have my thyroid checked. I have gained so much weight around the waist that perhaps it's my Cortisol.

A common concern of obese individuals that lead them to seek medical care is whether their obesity is "glandular," that is caused by a hormone abnormality. A number of endocrine (hormonal) changes accompany the obese state, most are secondary because they can be induced by overfeeding previously lean individuals and reversed with weight loss. Therefore, they are the result of obesity rather than the cause.

One key finding in obese, non-diabetic individuals is hyperinsulinemia (elevated blood insulin levels).[1] This correlates with the degree of obesity and is due to increase production of insulin by the pancreas. Despite the high levels of insulin, obese subjects do not become hypoglycemic (low blood sugar) suggesting that they may in fact be resistant to the action of insulin. Moreover, the degree of insulin resistance seems to depend on which action of insulin is being observed. Insulin resistance in obesity is greatest for blocking insulin's effect on carbohydrate metabolism by two actions: (1) reducing insulin's stimulation of glucose uptake by peripheral cells; and (2) by reducing the sensitivity to insulin's effect on suppressing hepatic(liver) glucose production. By blocking both of these actions insulin is prevented from lowering blood sugar, thereby leading to the development of 80% of the diabetics in the USA, who are usually overweight. These diabetics are usually referred to as type II or adult-onset.

One of the most requested and obtained tests for obesity is to check for hypothyroidism. The thyroid gland produces two thyroid hormones known as T_4 and T_3. The T_4 can be broken down inside cells to the more active T_3 form. Both of these hormones increase protein in virtually all body tissues, whereas, T_3 in addition increases

---

[1]Insulin plays a dominant and pivotal role in controlling glucose production and utilization. After feeding there is a rise in blood glucose from digestion which causes a surge of insulin from the pancreas to lower the blood glucose back to normal. High levels of insulin will reduce the body's production of glucose by inhibiting gluconeogensis and glycogenolysis, thereby reducing hepatic and renal glucose production. Peripheral glucose uptake and utilization in the peripheral tissues (including fat and muscles) are enhanced with lipolysis (breakdown of fat) and proteolysis (breakdown of protein) being restrained. Energy storage is promoted by the conversion of digested substrates into glycogen, triglycerides, and proteins. With caloric restriction and weight loss this process is reversed by low insulin levels. On the other hand glucagon is produced by the pancreas in response to a drop in blood glucose in order to restore the level by promoting glycogenolysis and gluconeogenesis.

metabolism in liver, kidneys, heart and skeletal muscle. Moreover, T_3 can be converted to relatively inactive form called rT_3 (reversed T_3). During reduced caloric intake such as "dieting or fasting", T_4 does not seem to change significantly whereas serum T_3 levels fall dramatically. There is an increase rT_3 during weight reduction secondary to decreased clearance (removal from blood by organs) and there is diversion of T_4 metabolism from T_3 to the less active rT_3. Supplementation of thyroid hormone during weight loss, to maintain a normal T_3 level has been associated with significant loss of protein (lean tissue or muscle) from 2 ½ to 9 times above non-fasting levels. Furthermore, thyroid supplementation on very low calorie diets had the greatest tendency for *curtailing* weight loss and was *paradoxically* associated with the lowest basal metabolic rate. For weight loss thyroid supplementation appears to be at the expense of loss of lean tissue over fat tissue and not recommended. Despite the drop in T_3, clinical hypothyroidism does not develop during weight loss.

The possibility of Cushing's syndrome (overproduction of cortisol in the body) is often an initial concern as the cause of obesity. Despite the common similarities of Cushing's Syndrome to obesity there is no evidence that obesity is associated with elevated cortisol levels. Although there is an increased production of cortisol in obesity there is a compensatory increase in the excretion in urine so that serum levels remain normal. The adrenal gland that produces cortisol, also, produces dihydroepiandosterone (DHEA) which is said to have anti-obesity effects in animals. Nevertheless, DHEA levels are normal in human obesity and administration of large doses to obese men produce no change in body weight.

There are low levels of testosterone (the predominate male hormone) in massively obese males with elevated levels of estrogen (female hormone) production, which are for the most part clinically silent and reversible by weight loss. However, the changes in sex hormones in women are interesting in that abdominal obesity (android) is associated with increased testosterone production with a higher incidence of menstrual disturbances and hirsutism (male pattern of hair growth) than in women with lower body fat (gynoid or predominant distribution in the hips and thighs). Also, android women have a high level of production of estrogen but is not elevated in gynoid women.[2] Weight loss reverses these abnormalities.

In addition to an elevated insulin level and low T_3 there is another consistent hormonal abnormality found in obesity: that is low levels of growth hormone. This low level of growth hormone is felt to be due to the high levels of insulin in obesity which suppresses growth hormone secretion. Although growth hormone levels are low, somatomedin (IGF-I) levels are normal. Growth hormone itself does not cause an effect, but, works by stimulating somatomedin which produces growth hormone's action. Therefore, obesity must result in a condition by which a lower amount of growth hormone can simulate enough somatomedin so that no physical evidence of a growth hormone deficiency state develops. During weight loss, fatty acids are increased with the breakdown of fat and insulin levels drop, both of which stimulate growth hormone secretion, thereby, reversing the low levels seen in obesity.

Overall the only significant hormonal change from endocrine glands present in obesity that contributes adversely to health is the overproduction of insulin by the pancreas. However, there is now substantial evidence that supports body weight being regulated by endocrine, metabolic and neural signals from the gut and fat cells. These signals are integrated by the hypothalamus of the brain for

[2]High levels of estrogen predispose these women to uterine and breast cancer.

control of appetite.[3] Although the fat cell (adipocyte) has long been regarded as a storage depot for fat, it is now clear that it is also an endocrine cell that can release numerous molecules that can affect other cells in a regulated fashion (this meets the definition of a hormone). Fat tissue (adipose tissue) is composed of the lipid storing adipocyte and, also, a protein vascular structure in which young un-evolved adipocytes reside. Adipose mass increases by enlargement of the adipose cell through fat deposition (as much as 20 times it original size) as well as by increasing a number of adipocytes (some 40 billion in an average adult up to 100 billion in some obese adults). Losing weight causes them to shrink in size and become less metabolically active, but their number goes down very slowly if at all.

Leptin is an adipocyte derived hormone (adipokine) that was first discovered in rodents and later found in humans (discussed in chapter 7). As adipose tissue increases so does the level of leptin in the blood, which informs the brain of the extent of adipose energy reserves. So, an increased amount of leptin, which informs the brain that there is plenty of fat available, is felt to suppress appetite and increase energy expenditure leading to weight loss. Leptin when administrated to genetically deficient rodents and some humans reverses obesity. However, absolute leptin deficiency in humans is a very rare cause of obesity. In fact, leptin levels are elevated in obese humans who seem to have developed a leptin resistance (similar to insulin resistance). During weight loss leptin levels drop lower than would be predicted by the decrease in fat. On the other hand, leptin increases proportionally as fat increases with no overshoot. Taken together, there may be an evolutionary reason for these differences of response .The primary role for leptin may be to indicate that fat

[3]The hypothalamus is that part of the brain just above the pituitary gland.

stores are sufficient for reproduction (leptin,also, promotes fertility). If levels of fat are low, so will be the level of leptin, thereby signaling increased appetite, low energy and a time to wait on reproducing. Therefore, if leptin is above a certain level it has little effect. This may be why obese humans with high leptin levels have neither increased appetite or increased energy expenditure. The Suppressor Of Cytokine Signaling 3 (SOCS 3) acts to limit the action of leptin signaling and is an important mediator of leptin resistance in the obese. Because SOCS 3, also, limits insulin singling, its expression provides a potentially important point of interaction between leptin and insulin pathways that may be important in the pathogenesis of the metabolic syndrome.[4]

There is further evidence that supports that body weight can be regulated by hormones from the gut by controlling appetite. Ghrelin is one such gut hormone (similar in structure to growth hormone) with appetite stimulation properties. Ghrelin activates neurons in the hypothalamus which increase NPY[5] and thereby appetite. Ghrelin is secreted predominately by the fundus (top part of the stomach) and also duodenum. Ghrelin levels rise during fasting and immediately before meals and fall quickly after eating suggesting a role of enhancing appetite and food intake. Ghrelin levels tend to be low in obese humans but increase with dietary weight loss thereby stimulating hunger. However, in obese individuals who undergo gastric bypass the blood levels of ghrelin do not peak in relation to meals and are markedly lower than both lean and obese subjects, despite the massive weight loss by the gastric bypass individuals. Therefore, whereas weight loss achieved by caloric restriction is

[4]The metabolic syndrome is associated with abdominal obesity, diabetes, hypertension and cholesterol abnormalities. Three of 5 of these problems together lead to an increased risk of coronary heart disease.
[5]Neuropeptide Y (NPY) is the most potent short-term stimulus for appetite.

associated with increased ghrelin levels in the blood, that achieved by gastric bypass is associated with abnormally low, non-oscillating levels. See Figure 8.1. This is consistent with post gastric bypass patients reporting less feelings of hunger. The reason for this discrepancy between diet and bypass is not known.

The gut is a source of numerous peptides (small proteins) that are involved with appetite and are referred to as incretin hormones. These are produced by single endocrine cells scattered throughout the intestines. Cholecystokinin (CCK) is produced by such cells in the duodenum and jejunum in response to food resulting in the reduction in meal size and inhibiting stomach emptying , thereby contributing to satiety.[6] Glucagon-like peptide (GLP-1) also inhibits stomach emptying and acid secretion, but, stimulates the endocrine pancreas to release insulin and to inhibit glucagon secretion after a meal. Glucose-dependent insulinotropic polypeptide (GIP) is stimulated by ingested fat and promotes its efficient storage into fat. Fasting levels of GIP are elevated and an exaggerated response to a meal is seen in the obese. Both of these are significantly reduced after gastric bypass. However, unlike ghrelin and GIP, CCK response to a meal is not altered by gastric bypass. Both GLP-1 and GIP are inactivated by an enzyme (DPP-4), which is itself blocked from inactivating these horomes by sitagliptin (a new diabetic medication) thereby causing an increase in insulin release and decreasing glucagon response to a meal leading to a lowering of the blood sugar, but at a cost of allowing GIP to promote fat storage.[7]

---

[6]CCK is also made in the brain (typeB). Since the anorectic effect is loss by vagotomy (cutting the nerve to the stomach) only the intestinal (type A) is mentioned here.

[7]Although the promotion of an insulin like effect by GIP is diminished with diabetes, GLP-1 continues to stimulate insulin secretion even in advance stages of diabetes.

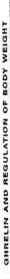

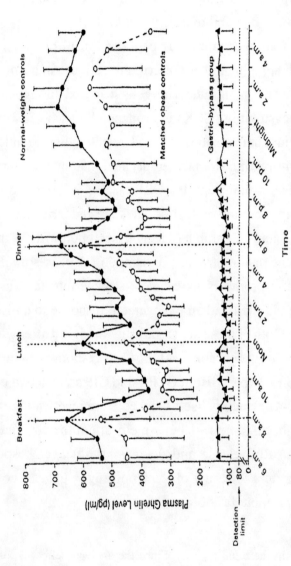

Fig. 8.1 The 24-hour plasma ghrelin levels in 5 obese subjects who underwent proximal Roux-en-Y gastric bypass (triangles), 5 obese subjects who had recently lost weight by diet (open circles), and 10 normal weight subjects with stable weight (closed circles). These subjects were matched according to final body mass index, age, and sex. Breakfast, lunch, and dinner were provided at times indicated. Cummings, DE, et al. (2002). Plasma ghrelin levels after diet-induced weight loss or gastric bypass surgery. *N Engl J Med, 346,* 1623-30. Reprinted with permission by the Massachusetts Medical Society, copyright 2002.

Besides such peptides, there are gut receptors that, when stimulated by contact with a specific substance, will unlock and set into motion a metabolic chain of events. One of these is the cannaboid receptor-1 which is not only found in the gut, but is found in the brain, muscle, and fat. When these receptors are stimulated, food intake and fat deposition is promoted. Recently, an antagonist (that which blocks the action) to the cannabinoid receptor-1 site has been shown to produce weight loss and ameliorate several other metabolic abnormalities associated with obesity including reducing abdominal girth and insulin resistance, while increasing good cholesterol (HDL) and adiponectin.[8]

In regards to hormones in obesity, two facts stand out that have produced insight into the control of appetite by the hypothalamus. Adenalectomy (removal of the adrenal glands where cortisol is produced) reverses or attenuates obesity. This can be seen in people with Addison's desease which is associated with adrenal insufficiency (low cortisol) and leanness, wheras, Cushing's syndrome (high cortisol) is associated with obesity. The other important finding pertains to prolactin which is made in the anterior pituitary gland to promote latation (milk production) in women. Prolactin release is under continuous inhibition by the hypothalamus, so that damage to the hypothalamus (loss of this inhibition) will lead to elevated

---

[8]Adiponectin is a cytokine (a protein involved in the regulation of the immune system and inflammation) from adipose tissue that reduces inflammation, increases insulin sensitivity (lowering blood sugar) and improves the balance of good (HDL) versus bad (LDL) cholesterol. Resistin is another cytokine made by fat that opposes adiponectin by contributing to insulin resistance. The fatter the person, the less adiponectin and more resistin is made. Internal (or visceral) fat produces more inflammatory (IL-6, TNF-alpha) and clot-promoting (PAI-1) factors than subcutaneous (just beneath the skin) fat. So, anything that reduces visceral fat is a good thing. Fortunately, visceral fat is the first to go with exercise. Unfortunately, it is not removed by liposuction – only subcutaneous fat is removed that way.

prolactin levels in the blood. Substances that increase prolactin output in normal weight subjects produce subnormal prolactin output in obese subjects and this reduced response persists after weight loss in obese subjects. This situation is in contrast to virtually all other instances of abnormal hormonal output in obesity in which the abnormalities are reversed by weight loss. This persistence of subnormal prolactin release in obese subjects, which is not corrected by weight loss, points to the possibility of an underlying hypothalamic dysfunction as an etiology of obesity.

Corticotrophin-releasing hormone (CRH) is a hypothalamic hormone that acts directly on the pituitary to increase the output of ACTH in the blood to stimulate cortisol production by the adrenal gland which then serves as a negative feedback as increased cortisol in the blood suppresses CRH. The paraventricular hypothalamus (PVH) is the site of the majority of CRH neurons projecting to the pituitary. This area receives input from the nucleus solitary tract, the gut, and from parts of the brain dealing with the perception of stress. CRH also acts on the hypothalamus to reduce food intake and stimulate sympathetic nervous system outflow (increase in energy use) causing sustained weight loss. Therefore, adrenalectomy reduces blood cortisol which in turn stimulates CRH which suppresses appetite and increases energy expenditure resulting in weight loss. On the other hand, the hypothalamus receives neuropojections from an area in the brain called the arcuate nucleus, which is relatively assessable to circulating factors in the blood. These attach to several areas of the hypothalamus including the paraventricular nucleus. Here, neuropeptide Y (NPY) stimulates food intake and lipoprotein lipase in the adipose tissue (which increases the uptake of fat cells) while inhibiting sympathetic nervous system outflow (thereby lowering energy expenditure). All of these changes by NPY promote weight gain. During weight loss low levels of leptin (decreased by reducing fat stores) and reduced levels of insulin stimulate NPY, as do high levels of cortisol, seen in other conditions.

Hormones from the gut and adipose tissue impinge on the arcuate nucleus of the brain which projects to the hypothalamus. Cortisol from the adrenals, as well as factors produced by physiological and psychological stresses, influence the hypothalamus directly through the blood. Together all these factors exert their effect to control appetite and energy expenditure from the hypothalamus. These two opposing factors struggle to achieve dominance to determine either an anabolic (weight gain) or catabolic (weight loss) course for the body. This is similar to the universal struggle of Yin/YANG. Fig. 8.2 Further research to either suppress adipocyte number, decrease NPY, or increase CRH (without increasing blood cortisol) appears most promising in regards to control of appetite.

Recognizing the hormonal changes that accompany obesity may prevent inappropriate treatments as well as provide new approaches to weight loss. The secondary nature of these hormonal changes due to obesity can be seen by the reversal of most following successful weight loss. Because there is a significant redundancy of both neural pathways and the hormones that affect appetite, a single therapeutic approach would most likely be overridden.[9] Lack of this knowledge has led many obese individuals to seek inappropriate treatment by purchasing pills that supposedly reverse hormones that cause obesity. None exist.

---

[9]Not only does the hypothalamus control appetite, but another part of the brain (hindbrain) can regulate food intake. Within the PP-fold peptide family of hormones, NPY stimulates appetite, whereas PYY and PP both reduce intake.

Fig. 8.2 The Yin/Yang of hypothalamic control of appetite

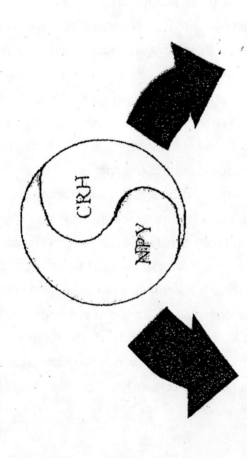

Anabolic (weight gain)
Increase food intake
Decrease energy output
Inhibited by insulin and leptin
Stimulated by cortisol

Catabolic (weight loss)
Decrease food intake
Increase energy output
Inhibited by cortisol
Stimulated by stress(psychological or
physiological)

Chapter 9
Mortality Muddled

Diary entry November 16th

A girl at the place where I work died yesterday. She was at least 300 pounds. I think this is God's way of telling me that I need to lose weight or I am going to die young.

Does intentional weight loss in overweight or obese individuals prolong life? The answer to this question is not as clear as one would imagine and is entangled with many dangers.

It is well known that obesity is associated with a modest increase in the relative risk of mortality, often in the range of 1.5 to 2. In many studies the graph of the relative risk of mortality as compared to the BMI follows a U or J-shaped curve. Please, refer to Figure 9.1. The minimum mortality is around a BMI of 25 with mortality increasing both as the BMI increases or decreases from 25. The highest mortality is at the extremes of either obesity or underweight. In reports from

Men

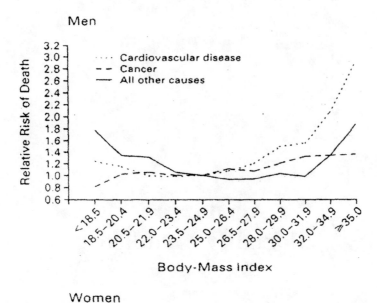

Women

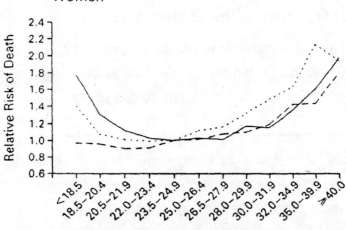

Fig. 9.1 The relative risk of death from cardiovascular disease, cancer, and all other causes according to Body Mass Index(BMI) among men and women who had never smoked and had no history of disease at enrollment. Calle,E.E. et al.(1999). Body-mass index and mortality in a prospective cohort of US adults. *N Engl J Med*, 341,1097-105. Copyright 1999, Massachusetts Medical Society. All rights reserved.Permission granted.

the National Health and Nutrition Examination Survey (NHANES)from 1971 through 2000 no increased mortality was associated with being overweight (BMI 25 to 30) even if overweight had persisted for at least 10 years. Furthermore, as compared to the earlier studies of NHANES I (1971-1975), the NHANES II (1976-1980) and the NHANES III (1988-1994), the impact of obesity on mortality has decreased over time. Improvements in medial care particularly for cardiovascular disease (leading cause of death among the obese) and its risk factors may have led to the decreased association of obesity with total mortality over this period of time. Cardiovascular risk factors have declined for all BMI categories in the U.S. population. Except for diabetes, the decline appears to be greater at the higher BMI levels. These findings are consistent with the increase in life expectancy in the U.S. and with the declining mortality rate in ischemic heart disease (heart attacks). Life expectancy increased from 74 years of age in 1980 to 75 years in 1990 to 77 years in 2000. Age adjusted death rates for ischemic heart disease declined from 345 per 100,000 in 1980 to 187 per 100,000 in the year 2000. All this has occurred while obesity rates have been climbing. In addition fitness has an impact on BMI and mortality relationship. *Unfit, lean* men had double risk of all cause mortality compared to *fit, obese* men. Also *unfit, lean* men had a higher risk of cardiovascular disease (heart, stroke and/or kidney vascular disease) mortality than did *fit, obese* men. Therefore, an active way of life appears to have important health benefits for those who are overweight/obese. However, *fit,obese* men without evidence of cardiovascular disease but with any one of the conditions that predispose to cardiovascular disease (diabetes mellitus, elevated cholesterol, hypertension, current cigarette smoking, low fitness) have about a 5 fold higher cardiovascular death rate and three fold higher all-cause death rate than *normal weight* men without any of these predisposing conditions.[1]

Similarly *overweight, but not obese*, men with one or more of the predisposed conditions have a three fold cardiovascular disease death rate and a two fold all-cause death rate than *normal weight* men without such conditions. These predisposing disease conditions are more likely with a high waist circumference (abdominal fat) and the association is greater in women than in men. In a study that adjusted out the risk of pre-existing diseases associated with excess weight, men with a BMI of 29 or more (*overweight or obese*) had a 30% reduction in cardiovascular disease/death with a weight loss of 5 to 14%. **This did not occur for women**. However, if these *obese* men lost greater than 15% of their body weight, the risk of death from cardiovascular disease was not reduced. Among *lean* men and women with BMI of 29 or less (normal to underweight) the risk of death increased with increasing weight loss. Among individuals who were *moderately overweight* (BMI of 26 to 29) those who lost 15% or more had more than twice the mortality risk from all-cause death than those without weight loss. So, if a man is overweight or obese, a little (5-14%) weight loss appears to be a good thing, but a big weight loss (more than 15%) may be a bad thing, and even worse for those who are overweight but not obese.

In women with an obesity related health condition(diabetes, high cholesterol, elevated blood pressure), intentional weight loss of any amount was associated with a statistically significant 20% reduction in all-cause mortality. This came not from decreased cardiovascular mortality, but was due to a significant (40 to 50%) reduction in

---

[1]Low fitness is of comparable importance to other cardiovascular disease risk factors as a strong independent predictor of mortality and cardiovascular disease death rates. However, fitness can be cancelled out by any one of the disease conditions that can be associated with obesity.

mortality from obesity related cancers (breast and uterine). Diabetes associated mortality was also significantly reduced by 30 to 40% in those women who intentionally lost weight. However, in women with no preexisting condition, intentional weight loss is not associated with any change in mortality.

There is evidence that suggests the highest mortality rates occur in adults who either have lost weight or gained excessive weight. Lowest mortality rates are generally associated with mild to moderate weight gain. People whose body weight fluctuates often or greatly have a higher risk of coronary heart disease and death than those with relatively stable body weight, independent of obesity and trend of body weight over time. Weight fluctuations most strongly associated with adverse health outcomes occur in the age group of 30 to 44 years of age, a time when dieting is likely to be most common. Body weight variability has been significantly correlated with a history of dieting (yo-yoing). Women age 55 to 69 years who have a large weight fluctuation (those who gained more than 10% of their body weight only to loose as much within the next measurement) had a higher incident of heart attack, stroke and diabetes as compared to those with stable or no weight change. Men 40 to 56 years of age who gained and lost weight over a 25 year period from 1958 to 1983 had a two fold increase in the relative risk of coronary death as compared to those with no change in weight. This was independent of their age, cholesterol, blood pressure, cigarette smoking status, alcohol intake or BMI.

Therefore, one may conclude that body weight variability (or voluntary weight loss with subsequent gain) is associated with a similar or higher risk of mortality and adverse health outcomes as those attributed to obesity. Plus, the risk due to excessive weight may not outweigh the risk due to weight fluctuation. However, what this really means is that overweight/obese individuals need to be taught skills to maintain weight loss and that prevention of relapse should become a more central focus of weight loss programs. Since exercise is effective in maintaining more than 75% of weight loss resulting from a weight reduction program, the long term benefits of weight loss would most likely occur through the increased cardiovascular fitness aspect and reduction of weight variability from the exercise required to maintain that reduced weight as discussed in chapter 4. This is consistent with studies that have shown that the probability of improved survival can be transferred from the unfit to those who become fit. See figure 9.2.

For more information on the effect of weight loss on the diseases associated with the overweight/obese, go to appendix IV. There is an even more surprising conclusion.

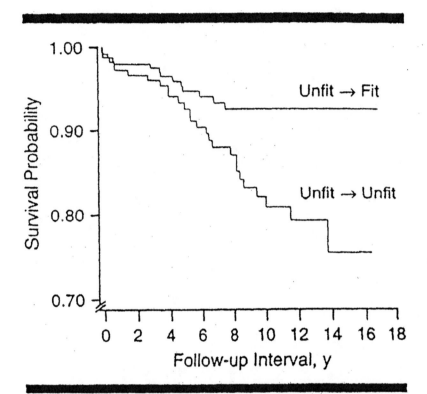

Fig. 9.2 Survival curves for change or lack of change in physical fitness in men revealing that unfit men who become fit improve their survival probability. Blair, Steven N., et al. (1995). Changes in physical fitness and all-cause mortality: a prospective study of healthy and unhealthy men. *JAMA*, 273, 1093-1098. Reprinted by permission from AMA, copyright 1995.

Chapter 10
Popular Diets Divulged

Diary Entry November 28th

There are so many diets to choose from. Which one is right? Is it carbs or fat that is the bad guy? Marge says she and her husband eat a pound of bacon everyday and are losing weight by avoiding carbs. Yet, everything at the grocery store has labels indicating lower fat is the way to go. Who is telling the truth?

The proliferation of books on weight loss has dramatically increased in the past six years.[1] Many different types of diet plans on the market are based on the macronutrient (fat, carbohydrate, protein) composition and range from low carbohydrate (high in fat and protein) to low fat (high in carbohydrate) with diets of a more lanced composition in between. Please refer to figure 10.1. As can

----

[1] A search on Amazon.com using the key word "weight loss" revealed 1214 matches in 2001 (Freedman, et al., 2001.). The same search in January of 2006 reveals 2607 matches.

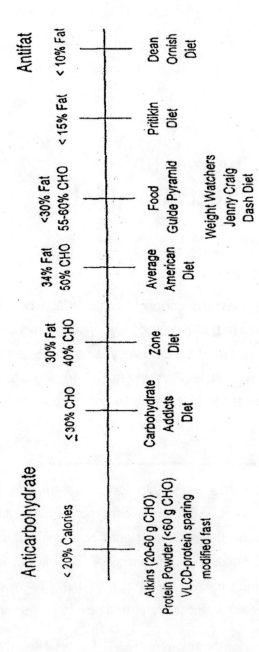

Fig. 10.1 The continuum of popularly known self-help diets ranging from anticarbohydrate (left) to antifat (right). CHO= carbohydrate. Riley, Rosemary E. (1999). Popular weight loss diets. *Clin Sports Med*, 18(3), 691-701. Reprinted with permission from Elsevier, copyright 1999.

be seen the average American diet falls somewhere in the middle of the two extremities (34% fat, 50% carbohydrate (CHO or carb), and 15% protein).

Those diets that advocate for low carbohydrate (Atkins®, Protein Power® and to a lesser extent the Zone® diet) do so to lower blood insulin which is looked upon as the root of the all metabolic ills of obesity. Except for Adkins diets, these diets focus on "good" and "bad" eicosanoids which are described as "powerful hormone like substances that control virtually all physiological functions in the body." To date none have been identified. In a recent study that compared *low carb*, high-fat diets to *high carb*, low-fat diets, both types of diets reduced insulin levels in the long term, except the Atkins in which it did not significantly change."The role of insulin in the synthesis and storage of fat has obscured its important effects in the central nervous system, where it acts to prevent weight gain, and has led to the misconception that insulin causes obesity." Insulin, also, has an indirect role in body weight regulation through stimulation of leptin. Both of these hormones (insulin and leptin) act to reduce hypothalamic neuropeptide Y(NPY) known to increase food intake and body weight. (See Chapter 8). Besides there are decreased or unchanged concentrations of insulin during weight loss regardless of the diet employed. Insulin, also, enhances the anorectic effects of cholecystokinin (CCK), often reputed to be the 'satiety hormone.' Obviously, simple explanations, especially ones that involve unknown substances are not the answer.

Nonetheless, much emphasis has been put on the macronutrient composition of diets used for weight loss. Many of the diets (on the left side of fig. 10.1) increase protein and fat while limiting the amount of carbohydrate. When carbohydrate consumption is less than 40 grams per day, the body shifts into a metabolic state of using ketones and fatty acids from the breakdown of fat (ketosis) as its major source for energy. (See Chapter 5). This would imply fat loss through reduced carbohydrate consumption. However, in a recent systematic review of published studies using low-carbohydrate diets which varied significantly in calories from carbs, weight loss while using low-carbohydrate diets (less than 60 grams/day) was principally associated with decreased caloric intake and increased diet duration, but not with the reduction of carbohydrate content as no difference in weight loss was found using a higher or lower carb diet. Furthermore, studies have been done in which obese patients were placed on the same low calorie diet, but the proportion of carbohydrate was varied. One would suspect then that there would be variable weight loss in that the lowest carbohydrate diet would lose more than the high content diet if carbohydrates influenced fat loss. However, weight loss was the same for all. Therefore, carbohydrate macronutrient composition does not play a major role in weight loss, but it is caloric restriction that is the major determinant. A similar finding was found in a comparison of Aitkin's®, Ornish®, Weight Watchers® and Zone® diets for weight loss in which there was no significant differences in weight loss between the diets no matter which macronutrient (fat vs. carbohydrate) was restricted. Also, for each diet, there was a decrease in cardiac risk factors of lower total/HDL cholesterol, C-reactive protein (an inflammation marker), and lower insulin level that were significantly associated with the weight loss, but no significant difference with which diet was consumed. Nonetheless, an important observation should be made in regards to diet composition. The low carbohydrate diets were unrestricted to the amount of calories eaten, while in most studies the high carbohydrate (low fat) dieters were, also, instructed on caloric restriction. Yet weight loss was usually the same. The fact is that the low-carbohydrate-diet participants voluntarily eat fewer calories.

Diets recommended by various national health organizations for chronic disease prevention are low in fat and high in carbohydrate. In fact, the original recommendation to reduce fat in the diet (the foundation of these present day national guidelines) was introduced in 1970 as a means of lowering serum cholesterol for the prevention of heart disease and were later on adopted by the American Medical Association. Obviously, these recommendations were not enough to prevent the recent rise in obesity and diabetes (each alone an independent risk factor for heart disease). In the Seven Countries Study which investigated the relationship between diet and heart disease, Crete, which had the lowest incidence of heart disease, had a high total fat intake of 40% of the food eaten per day. In the Netherlands, which has a high life expectancy and lowest obesity prevalence in Europe, fat made up 48% of the total diet. Recently the Harvard School of Public Heath which had originally suggested that fat intake may play a role in obesity, has now proposed that reducing the percent of fat in the diet will have no important benefits on obesity and could further exacerbate the problem. Furthermore, the emphasis on fat reduction has been a serious distraction in efforts to control obesity. The NHLBI states "there is little evidence that lower-fat diets cause weight loss independent of calorie restriction." Obese individuals, who consume diets of the same amount of calories, but containing different amounts of calories from fat (15%-34%), for 12 weeks will lose the same amount of weight.

Other diets have sought different creative means to cause weight loss. These include the Glycemic Index, Energy Density, and high fiber plans discussed next. These diets are aimed at creating decreased feelings of hunger (increase satiety). But, as we have seen in chapter

1, hunger is more often due to psychological stress rather than an actual physiologic need to sustain energy stores.

The glycemic index (GI) has been endorsed by the Food and Agriculture Organization of the World Health Organization for weight control in the obese. Compared with low-GI meals, high GI meals induce a greater rise and fall in blood glucose and with the resultant greater rise in blood insulin there is a lowering of the concentrations of the body's two main fuels (blood glucose and fatty acids) in the immediate post-digestive period. It is proposed that the reduced availability of metabolic fuels may act as a signal to stimulate more eating. However, there are no long term studies that support using low-GI diets in the prevention or treatment of obesity. In one study the rate of glucose appearance was the same for a low-GI cereal as for one that had a GI that was twice as high, and the amount of insulin response was similar. It appears that the low-GI cereal had 3.5 times more protein, which probably explained the rapid insulin response and attenuated glycemic response. Therefore, other factors (such as protein or fat) in the diet may play a more important role or interaction with the GI so as to affect its response.

In general the human body weight remains fairly constant for prolonged periods of time with about 2/3 of the day-to-day fluxuations within 0.5 percent and 1/3 within 1.5 percent of total body weight. Despite such relative stability of body weight, there is little evidence for a fine temporal adjustment of energy regulation between the energy expended and the caloric intake on any one day. When the caloric concentration of meals is diluted without knowledge of the *lean* individual, more volume or weight of food is consumed to meet the caloric needs to maintain their weight. However, *obese* subjects fail to sense the drop in energy density and continue to consume the same volume or weight of food with resultant weight loss due to the fewer calories consumed. The major determinants of dietary *energy density* (ED)[2] are water and fat with ED falling as water content rises and as fat content falls. Protein and carbohydrates contribute relatively little to ED. Therefore, following ED of food is equivalent to following a low fat diet.

Nonetheless, some investigators feel that the amount (weight or volume) of food consumed, independent of its energy content, can subsequently effect the amount of food eaten. In one such study men were given food of different volumes of equal energy content and macronutrients (casserole versus soup made from that casserole) before lunch. Those who consumed the larger volume (soup) ate less not only for lunch, but also at the following evening meal. Certainly, decreasing the energy density of and increasing the volume of a premeal (that which is eaten before a meal) by adding water to it can increase fullness, reduce hunger and subsequent energy intake in the short term. However, simply drinking water either before or with a meal has no effect on food intake. Another means of decreasing energy density is to add fiber which for the most part is not digested to provide energy. Furthermore, fiber tends to bind water leading to an additional lowering of the energy density of the food. When there is no restriction on the amount of food eaten, the consumption of an additional 14 grams/day of fiber for more than 2 days/week is associated with a 10% decrease in energy intake (calories) and body weight loss of 4 pounds over 4 months.

Therefore, caloric restriction rather than macronutrient composition is the major determinant of weight loss. The average American consumes 2200 calories a day.[3] As shown in Table 10.1,

[2]The ED can be defined as the energy (calories) per mass of the food (calories per gram). Low ED foods are less than 1.5 and high ED foods are greater than 4.0.

[3] A very conservative estimate is 2860 calories/day for an individual younger than 50 years who weighs 220lbs with a sedentary lifestyle.

individuals who lost weight in the National Weight Control Registry (NWCR) reduced their caloric intake significantly (1300 calories/d for women and 1800 calories/d for men) with only a slight reduction of fat (from 35% to 24%). Table 10.2 compares the NWCR weight maintenance diet (bottom line) to the macronutrient composition of other popular diets. The NWCR *maintenance* diet most closely resembles the moderate-fat, balanced nutrient *reduction* diet.[4] Once again, even in reduced-obese individuals calorie restriction remains more important than the macronutrient composition of the diet in maintaining their new weight.

---

[4] Note that the 1570 calories/day eaten by weight maintainers of the NWCR is lower than the average of 2200 calories/day of the average American diet. See Chapter 2.

Dietary intakes of National Weight Control Registry enrollees by method of weight loss

Nutrient	Women (number)		Men (number)	
	On own (128)	With assistance (227)	On own (46)	With assistance (37)
Calories	1336 ± 494	1289 ± 443	1809 ± 733	1531 ± 478
Protein (%)	18.1 ± 3.3	19.9 ± 3.8	17.5 ± 4.3	19.1 ± 3.4
CHO (%)	55.9 ± 10.7	55.2 ± 8.4	55.5 ± 8.8	57.1 ± 8.1
Fat (%)	24.8 ± 9.6	24.0 ± 7.2	24.1 ± 8.5	22.8 ± 6.8

Table 10.1 The dietary intakes of the National Weight Loss Control Registry enrollees by method of weight loss. The average American diet consists of 2200 cal/day with 34% from fat and 50% from carbohydrates(CHO). Freedman, Marjorie R., King,J., and Kennedy, E. (2001). Popular diets: a scientific review. *Obesity Research*, 9(suppl.1), 1S-40S. Permission granted by NAASO, The Obesity Society, copyright 2001.

Characterization of diets used for weight loss and weight maintenance

Type of diet	Total kcals	Fat g (%)	CHO g (%)	Protein g (%)
High-fat, low-CHO*	1450	97 (60)	36 (10)	108 (30)
Moderate-fat, balanced nutrient reduction	1450	40 (25)	218 (60)	54 (15)
Low- and very-low-fat	1450	16–24 (10–15)	235–271 (65–75)	54–72 (15–20)
Weight maintenance	1491	40 (23.9)	208 (55.9)	72 (19.2)

* Based on average intake of subjects who self-selected low-CHO diets; studies lasting more than one week.

Table 10.2 Characterization of diets used for weight loss and maintenance. The last line represents the diet consumed by individuals in the National Weight Control Registry, who have maintained a 30 pound weight loss for at least 5 years. Freedman, Marjorie R., King,J., Kennedy,E. (2001). Popular diets: a scientific review. Obesity Research, 9(suppl 1), 1S–40S. Permission granted by NAASO, The Obesity Society, copyright 2001.

Chapter 11
Conclusion: Terrible Two's

Al Gore, former vice-president of the USA, in the documentary film, An Inconvenient Truth, said: "I have seen scientists who were persecuted, ridiculed, and deprived of jobs/income simply because the facts they discovered led to an inconvenient truth that they insisted on telling."

Many obese individuals have a history of childhood abuse (sexual, mental or physical) that has led to what is called learned helplessness. This in turn has led to the high levels of mood disorder (depression and anxiety) seen in the overweight/obese population. These moods lead to negative assumptions about the self with a sense of vulnerability developing. This in turn sets up what is referred to as despair behavior. Initially, there is a denial, followed by anger (usually turned inward), resulting in repeated failures that feed back into the learned helplessness state. The longer this occurs, the easier it is to provoke and the harder it is to stop. Without a behavioral approach to weight loss, many reduced individuals are not equipped to handle these and many others flaws that were once blamed on obesity. These individuals are doomed to failure as has become common place with the current approach. These issues must be addressed during and after the weight loss phase.

Not only do psychological issues persist after weight loss, but physical changes induced by weight loss persists for many years afterwards. The reduction of metabolism during weight loss can persist for six years, meaning that the reduced-obese individual has to make a life long commitment to daily regulation of diet and exercise. The new diet needs to average 1000 calories less than others at the same weight who have not been obese, and based on adherence to new behavioral changes in coping with social and personal stressors. A daily exercise program that is equal in one day to that recommended for non-reduced people for a week must be maintained indefinitely. Therefore, obesity must be thought of as a chronic disease, yet less than half (42%) of physicians recently polled believe that obesity is a disease.[1] Obviously, many obese individuals are not given the support they need.

In current medically supervised weight-loss programs rapid weight loss has been thought to lead to rapid loss of active muscle and strength, and therefore, discouraged. But, many studies do not demonstrate the loss of strength or endurance with diet/exercise plans. Post-gastric bypass patients loose 3 for 4 times faster than those on conventional diets. Why does it appear appropriate to do so surgically, but not medically? Frustrated, more obese individuals look to blame genetics or hormones for their weight. Although there is a small genetic component, it is for the most part latent and of little impact, being induced by excessive food intake and lack of

---

[1] What is even more disturbing is that 95% of physicians in this study discuss diet and exercise with their obese patients and 95% feel that there are effective treatments for obesity, but 95% never or rarely prescribe medications for weight loss.

physical activity. The high levels of insulin appear as a consequence of obesity and not the cause, as do most all hormonal abnormalities seen in obesity, and are for the most part reversed by weight loss. In desperation many seek a quick fix through surgery, fad diets or pills.

There are no quick fixes. The treatment of obesity is a life long process of changing not only eating habits, but developing and continuing physical activity on a daily basis. Weight loss is achieved by reducing food intake, but that should not be a goal in itself. Maintenance through *daily exercise* and a *reduced diet* (*the terrible two's*) in order to avoid weight fluctuations (yo-yoing) is critical. These weight loss/gain episodes are deadly and associated with a similar or higher risk of mortality and adverse health outcomes as those attributed to those who remain obese. Therefore, medical treatment and supervision of weight loss by diet/exercise programs or by surgery need to be continued for a lifetime, much as with the treatment of hypertension.

The myths that have evolved around weight loss are so perverse, that a whole dogma has developed around them. Many in the medical community have come to accept them as unquestionable truths. Even with the scientific evidence as presented here, the more informed and forward thinking physicians have been met with skepticism and ridicule by many in the medical community who are not willing to question the status quo and have gone to great lengths to discredit their work, even when faced with their successful results. It is by exposing these myths, that effective weight loss programs can be developed. Often, it is seen that individuals exhaust themselves by over exercising to lose weight only to be frustrated time and time again not realizing the scientific evidence against losing weight by exercise alone. Furthermore, with a concentrated devotion to counting food and/or use of food substitutes as advocated by many weight loss programs, attention is misdirected from the underlying psychological issues that need to be addressed to prevent relapse.

First, by exposing these myths through scientific evidence can the ineffectiveness of medically supervised weight loss programs be overcome. It is the dogmatic belief in these myths by many uninformed physicians that have left most overweight/obese individuals helplessly stranded with the only alternative left to them but to turn to those who take advantage of their desperation by selling fads and gimmicks with no (or misleading) scientific basis. This has allowed the creation of a multi-billion dollar a year industry that has helped fuel the obesity epidemic in this country by proposing deceptive, and misleading claims of effectiveness protected by freedom of speech. Often major advances in medicine are often met with derision not only by those who are uninformed or misinformed, but by those who stand to lose a great deal of money or status by change.

Using the scientific facts presented here, I have had a successful weight loss program for the past twelve years in which 90% of my time is spent with the patient in dispelling myths. Often it takes a leap of faith driven by years of frustration. It is hoped that the data presented here will initiate a paradigm shift in current weight loss management so that scientific knowledge that has been available for many years (decades) can be applied to wipe out the current state of deceptive and misinformed manipulation of the public. Such a weight loss program that incorporates the evidence-based facts presented in this text into a successful weight loss and maintenance program has been the basis of my success and will be discussed in detail in my next book.

Appendix I
From shocking dogs to frightening babies — a theory develops

Psychoanalytic theories have assumed that overeating in the overweight/obese individual is a maladaptive coping response to depression and anxiety. In a study of obese individuals applying for a weight loss program, almost half had major depression or an anxiety disorder. But, what has caused this behavior of overeating? What is the cause of this coping response?

In regards to depression and anxiety, cognitive theory has come into favor in recent years, involving the concept of *learned helplessness*. The animal model of learned helplessness has been extensively studied for more than 30 years. In the original experimental study, dogs were placed in a box in which they received electric shocks through a grid in the floor. They could avoid the shocks by going to the other side of the box. Not surprisingly, the dogs learned to terminate the shocks rather quickly by moving to the other side. However, when the situation was changed so that the dogs could not escape the shock, the dogs tended to lie down and accept the shocks passively. In this situation even when the barrier preventing the animal from escaping the shock was removed, the dogs continued to act as though they could not get away. The dogs could not be coxed away from the shock; only forcibly dragging the dog to safety could the painful shocks be terminated. The interpretation of this was that the inescapable shock they had experienced earlier had become imprinted so as to make them unable to cope even when there was a change that allowed control. In other words they learned to be helpless. It took many efforts of forcibly dragging the dogs across the barrier for them to finally learn that they could escape. This would imply that an outside force could change this learned behavior, but it would take persistence.

In regards to depression and anxiety negative thinking appears to be the cause rather than the result of both. Early experiences lead to the development of negative assumptions (schemata). Depressive schemata usually involve all or nothing assumptions such as:

1) If I am not completely happy then I will be totally miserable.
2) If I am not in complete control then I am helpless.
3) If I depend on anyone then I am totally needy.

Depression in this model results from experiences of failure to control events. These result in feelings of helplessness and hopelessness which eventually develop into generalized expectation of failure and inadequacy. There develops a deep sense of worthlessness and inadequacy through repeated experiences of feeling weak, unprotected, and unable to cope. Experiences of loss and abandonment produce a dependent type of depression, whereas, experience of invalidation produce a self-critical depression.

Anxiety is both a biologic (a fear reaction) and a learned (or conditioned) response. The first demonstration that human fears can be conditioned was done in 1920 on an 11 month old child named Little Albert. The patient was shown a white rat contiguous with a loud noise producing a frightened response from little Albert. Eventually just the white rat alone produced a fear reaction in Little Albert. By avoiding the fear stimulus to reduce the tension, avoidance behavior is reinforced in situations that produce anxiety, which is mediated by the individual's experiences and expectations. There is a sense of uncontrollability regarding future threats. Now anxiety is conceived of as a product of danger related schemata stored in the memory through painful life experiences. The anxiety state is associated with helplessness that results in one's inability to predict or control outcomes, characterized prominently by negative evaluation of one's ability to cope.

A sense of vulnerability in depression and anxiety leads individuals to interpret failures and deficiencies as a chronic inability to cope with unpredictable and uncontrollable events. The continued or repeated avoidance of the perceived threat allows feelings of depression and anxiety to become ingrained. This withdrawal elicits negative input from others which reinforces feelings of helplessness and solidifies the individuals identity as someone unfulfilled, overwhelmed and incompetent. As more time is spent in these mood states remissions are less complete and new recurrences develop with less provocation. The episodes are more likely to become more abrupt, more severe and more complex in their expression. In this way the individual learns to become helpless much as in the dog experiments noted above. Figure 1 outlines this cognitive concept of how learned helplessness influences eating disorders. Repeated trauma either sexually, physically or mentally from which there is no escape is

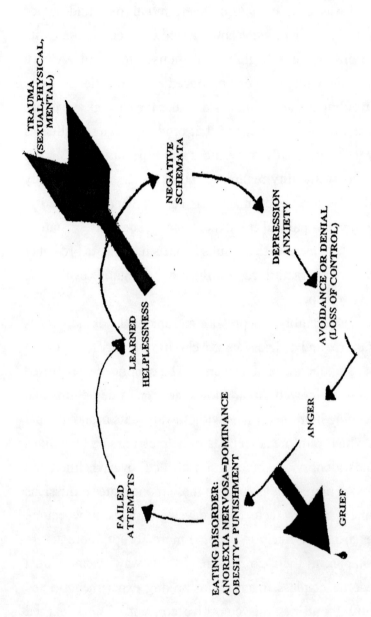

FIGURE 1) COGNITIVE MODEL FOR EATING DISORDERS:

The wounded heart was chosen for this model for various reasons, The entry wound is small and, often, quite hard to find. Many times individuals lack insight into the etiology of their negative beliefs about themselves. The exit wound is often large and produces most of the damage. The grief reaction of initial denial then attempts at resolution often create this obvious exit wound, often the initiating event. This usually occurs in childhood which is the most vulnerable time of life. This leads to learned helplessness or despair behavior. Learned helplessness produces negative schemata, which leads to depression and/or anxiety. These stages lead to a grief reaction in which initially avoidance or denial of the loss of control is encountered. This can lead to a state of anger or rage which is turned in on one's self. This can be expressed as an eating disorder. In anorexia nervosa the anger is directed more at control for a sense of empowerment, whereas, in obesity anger is in the form of punishment for low self-esteem. Attempts at changing this maladaptive eating behavior is often met with failures which then reinforces the negative schemata and learned helplessness of previous traumas. By directing the attention only to the eating disorder and not to the initiating traumatic events that produce learned helplessness, many weight loss programs are domed to failure.

Weight loss programs must include behavior treatment for learned helplessness to be successful. Special attention has to be paid to positive reward conditioning, social skills and structured problem solving therapies. Each positive experience should reinforce the feeling of accomplishment and self worth. Therefore, behavior therapy must be an integrate part at the start as well as during the maintenance of weight loss programs.

Appendix II
Children are born with innate fear of water, not food selection

In the 1920's and 1930's the pediatrician Clara Davis conducted studies on diet selection by infants and young children. During the first quarter of the 20th century most infants were not given solid food until they were nearly a year old and then the transition from suckling to a diet of food eaten by adults would be made gradually over a three to four year period. This is in stark contrast to present day recommendations that solid foods be introduced into an infant's diet between the ages of 4 and 6 months. The research by Dr. Davis focused on identifying the foods the infants would in the absence of adult intervention select to eat and in determining whether the food in the amount selected would be adequate to maintain growth and digestive health. What Dr. Davis found was that infants selected a combination of foods in quantities sufficient for growth. The diet selection consisted only of fresh unprocessed food, un-sweated and prepared simply and without combinations. All infants had a low preference for all ten vegetable groups offered. Milk intake accounted for 40% of total calories supplied and 70% of the Recommended Daily Allowance (RDA) nutrients except iron which was below the RDA recommendation amount. The most common misinterpretation of these results led to the myth that infants and children have an innate ability to select a balanced nutritious diet for themselves. The subjects of Dr. Davis had no access to sweats or junk foods and so they did not have to wrestle with temptation. The primary conclusion from her research was that solid foods could be eaten by infants and young children and their appetite was a reliable guide for the amount of food, "not the nutritional quality". This was also confirmed by a resent study in 1991. One has to take into account that food intake in humans increases as the variety of foods offered at a meal increases. Therefore, the restriction of food selection rather than innate ability to select needed foods was responsible for the dietary adequacy observed. Furthermore, it has long been observed that animals fed standard laboratory rations would not overeat and would not become obese even when food was overly abundant, but obesity can be easily produced in laboratory rats by giving unlimited access to a highly palatable "supermarket diet" of chocolate chip cookies, marshmallows, milk chocolate, salami, peanut butter and cheese. Therefore, deciding how much food to consume should be the purgative of the child. However, the selection of the diet should be balanced and nutritious made by the parents and not offered to reward or punish certain kinds of behavior.

Appendix III
Exercise : the Metabolic Paradox

Skeletal muscle contains only a very limited amount of stored energy in the form of glycogen. This is less energy than would be needed in a 100 yard dash, or about 10 seconds of intense exercise. Therefore, muscle must obtain energy for even a limited amount of work from outside sources. Two fuels are available to skeletal muscle for this purpose: 1) blood glucose mainly from the breakdown of liver glycogen 2) free fatty acids (FFA) derived from fat. However, the glycogen from the liver is in short supply, too, and would provide enough energy to sustain running for only six miles, while fat (adipose tissue) could possibly provide enough energy to run from Boston to Atlanta for an average weight person. At rest and during intense exercise skeletal muscle utilizes both free fatty acids (FFA) and glycogen for energy.[1] As exercise begins the enzyme, lipoprotein lipase(LPL), is stimulated to breakdown triglycerides in fat and muscle cells to glycerol and FFA. These FFA enter the muscle cell where the comparatively few mitochondria metabolize

[1]Skeletal muscle accounts for 20-30% of the body's energy expenditure at rest and up to 90% during exercise. At rest more than 80% of the muscle's energy is supplied by fat.

them for energy in the presence of an adequate oxygen supply. As the intensity of exercise increases and outstrips the supply of oxygen the utilization of FFA declines, and glycogen stored in the muscle becomes more important and at maximum work the muscle depends entirely on glycogen. This shift to glycogen is due to the fact that glycogen consumes less oxygen than fat to produce the same amount of energy. As a result there is a shift from aerobic metabolism (when oxygen is available) of FFA with CO_2 and water as by-products to anaerobic (where oxygen is limited) metabolism of glucose (stored as glycogen) resulting in the build up of lactate (lactic acid) which limits muscular performance and produces the muscle aches that follow strenuous exercise.[2] Therefore, every effort must be made to spare the breakdown of muscle glycogen. Blood glucose, then, becomes important with exercise lasting more than 20 minutes. There is an increase in the output of glucose from the liver and an enhancement of glucose uptake by the muscle during this time. As a result blood glucose can supply as much as 30% of the metabolic needs of exercising muscle thus sparing muscle glycogen to some extent. There is a capacity to increase free fatty acid utilization with repeated, prolonged exercise(endurance training) through increased intramuscular triglyceride storage and increased activity of LPL in adipose and muscle tissues.

Also, there is good evidence that an individual's ability to sustain prolonged exercise is highly dependent on the glycogen content of the muscles which in turn, can be dependent on the type of diet before exercise. During exhaustive exercise muscle glycogen content can be almost completely emptied. If a high fat/protein, low carbohydrate diet is followed after such exercise, only a slow, incomplete resynthesis

---

[2]The point at which lactic acid appears in the blood is referred to as the anaerobic threshold or maximum aerobic capacity. See Chapter 4.

of glycogen takes place. If a high carbohydrate diet is given after exhaustive exercise, there is enhanced glycogen synthesis with complete restoration of pre-exercise levels in the muscles that have been exhausted and not others. This restoration can occur within 24 hours post exercise and additional glycogen can be synthesized over the next few days. With higher initial glycogen concentration, the muscle's ability to sustain prolonged exercise is increased.

The changes in the metabolism of exercising skeletal muscle are modulated by a number of hormonal changes. One of which is a fall in insulin levels. This, along with other changes, creates a tendency to elevate blood glucose. Glucose ingested during exercise tends to maintain blood glucose levels; however, ingestion of glucose before exercise may actually raise insulin levels and thereby block energy mobilization. Contrary to popular belief pre-exercise meals or power drinks should not contain concentrated sweets, in fact, little other than water should be drunk two hours before exercise to prevent an elevation of insulin.

In recent years, there have been many dietary supplements that claim to boost fat metabolism, reduce fat, and improve athletic performance. The ability to enhance fat metabolism while conserving endogenous carbohydrate stores is the ultimate goal to prolonging exercise. As muscle and liver glycogen become depleted, fatigue begins. Caffeine has both a glycogen sparing effect and a positive effect on fat metabolism. In amounts of 150 to 250 mg caffeine can improve performance in continuous, moderate-intensity exercise. Therefore, caffeine can improve duration of exercise at a 65% maximum effort, where fat breakdown is at its highest level. This intensity of exercise induces a progressive mobilization of fatty acids from the adipocytes into the blood stream. However, at high doses caffeine can produce hypertension, irritability, detrimental changes in heart rate, and other adverse events.

Many dietary supplements that promote themselves as inducing weight loss contain caffeine. A popular product contains an extract from the rind of the brindall berry – hydroxycitric acid (HCA). In two human clinical studies when HCA was compared to placebo (a pill containing no active ingredient), no difference was found in weight loss. However, many such products contain caffeine, which is most likely the effective factor in such mixtures. But, as discussed above, caffeine facilitates metabolic changes that enable muscle to work longer, not to promote weight loss by itself. If the results of these changes are not utilized, then the energy is restored as fat. Even with exercise, there appears to be a redistribution and repackaging of fat so that even highly trained athletes with little adipose tissue have fat stores that far exceed their athletic needs. Endurance athletes have small but significant amounts of triglyceride stored as droplets within the muscle cell that are not seen in the untrained. These physiologically important changes can be quickly lost.[3]

Although a number of exercise programs infer that they can increase metabolism during weight loss and thereby increase weight loss, the evidence is lacking. Although a few studies show a 5 to 19% higher RMR per muscle mass in highly active individuals over sedentary ones, this requires months to years to achieve and only days to lose. This should be interpreted with caution because of genetic differences, degree of adaptation to training and nutritional status. In carefully controlled endurance training studies lasting from 3 to 12 weeks, no improvement in RMR measured 36 to 72 hours

---

[3]The best overall measurement of training effect, cardiovascular fitness, or physical fitness is the maximal oxygen uptake (VO_{2MAX}). Just 3 weeks of bed rest will cause a 20% to 25% decline in VO_{2MAX}. In contrast, regular training of weeks or months will improve VO_{2MAX} by about 30 to 40%. See chapter 3.

after last exercise bout was found in either lean or obese subjects. In some studies that demonstrated an increase in RMR, food intake was not measured or weight gain occurred, both of which are associated with a higher RMR. Most studies that showed improvement in RMR with training also showed a rapid drop off of the RMR after 15 hours. There appears to be a fast and slow component of recovery back to baseline RMR after exercise. First, there is a fast drop in the oxygen consumption (VO_2) over 2 to 10 minutes, followed by a slow drop back to the pre-exercise level over the next 2 hours.[4] Therefore, one can obtain discordant results for RMR depending on the time post exercise. Also, the intensity of exercise can effect RMR. When exercise is performed at 35-68% of maximal capacity for 20 to 80 minutes, the RMR is elevated for a short time (minutes) and rapidly recovers to the pre-exercise level. However, if exercise is done at 50-78 % VO_{2max} for 80 to 180 minutes on a regular basis (weeks to months), the RMR can be 5-20% elevated at 2.5 to 12 hours after exercise. Most of these elevations of metabolic rate are not sustained beyond 24 hours, unless done on a regular basis for years. Therefore, these observations indicate that there is an intensity-duration threshold for exercise to produce a prolonged effect on metabolism. As discussed in chapter 2, this all changes when weight loss is added. There appears to be a paradoxical drop in the metabolic rate during dietary weight loss when exercise is added that exceeds those who do not exercise. Dieters who add a 50% VO_{2max} exercise program (which increases VO_{2max} in non-dieters allowed free access to food) to a very low calorie diet develop a metabolic rate that can be 17% below those on the same diet who choose not to exercise. This is supported by another study showing a 17% reduction in resting metabolism

[4]There is a linear relationship between VO_2 and RMR (resting metabolic rate), so that as one increases so does the other, visa versa. At times it may be easier to measure VO_2 rather than RMR.

in soldiers performing daily exercise while on a similar restricted diet.

Furthermore, exercise metabolism is the dynamic interaction of muscle and body fat that not only changes during exercise, but somehow afterwards. Whereas at high intensity exercise, energy is derived mainly from carbohydrate (breakdown of glycogen), in contrast, low intensity exercise derives energy from the breakdown products of fat. If exercise contributed significantly to weight loss, then one would expect a difference to occur by varying the intensity. As discussed in chapter 3, exercise does not contribute to any consequential increase in weight loss or preferential fat loss when added to diet. Certainly, after exercise there is a redistribution of energy to restore the imbalances brought about by exercise. There, also, appears to be an obligatory drop in metabolism exacerbated by exercise during weight loss negating any benefit. Each of these is a paradox. Furthermore, caffeine's effect of improving metabolism is not associated with any evidence of increased fat breakdown, and therefore, caffeine's benefit may be in its ability to improve endurance performance, and thereby, better adherence to a routine exercise program, rather than its metabolic action. Since low intensity exercise is better tolerated by the obese, it would be the choice of exercise based on better compliance to be continued in the maintenance phase of weight loss. Exercise becomes of major importance in the reduced-obese individual after weight stabilization, where the exercise paradox induced during weight loss is no longer present.

Appendix IV
Disease Burden of Obesity-Stain or Stigma

In 1991 the estimated number of annual deaths due to obesity among U.S. adults was about 280,000. By 2000 it was estimated to be 400,000. It is well established that obesity is associated with a substantial burden of disease. Obesity accounts for about 90 to 95% of all diagnosed cases of diabetes mellitus in the United States and the risk for development of diabetes increases dramatically as the weight increases. The increase in hypertension (elevated blood pressure) begins at relatively low levels of weight gain. There is evidence that being overweight is a predictor of coronary heart disease (CHD) independent of its effects on hypertension, cholesterol and blood sugar. There is a 72% increase in risk of fatal or non-fatal coronary heart disease (CHD) of middle aged men with a BMI of 25 to 29 compared to men having BMI of less than 23. As a result the American Heart Association has added obesity to its list of major risk factors for the development of CHD. Obesity has been identified as a predisposing factor for hypoventilatory and obstructive *sleep apnea*, which is the cessation of breathing during sleep for at least ten seconds.[1] One study showed that the risk for ischemic stroke (due to lack of blood flow) was 75% higher in women with BMI of greater than 27 and 137% higher in those with BMI greater than 32 as compared to those with BMI of less than 21. The risk for gall stones and cholecystecotmy (removal of gall bladder) increases with weight gain. Non-alcoholic steatohepatits (NASH) is a fatty infiltration of the liver associated with inflammation of fibrosis as seen in alcoholic liver disease but occurs mostly in overweight individuals who do not drink alcohol excessively. With sustained weight loss there is resolution of NASH. Increased body weight has, also, been shown to increase the risk of disabling knee osteoarthritis and gout.

The metabolic syndrome is a constellation of cholesterol and non-cholesterol risk factors of metabolic origin linked to insulin resistance in which the normal actions of insulin are impaired. In total, three out of five risk factors (one of which is abdominal obesity) will enhance the risk of coronary heart disease regardless of the level of cholesterol. Most studies clearly show an increase in mortality rate associated with a BMI of at least 30 in the range of 50% to 100% increase risk (double the rate) from death due to all causes compared to those with a BMI of 20 to 25. Most of the increase in mortality is due to cardiovascular causes, such as, heart attack, hypertension or renal vascular disease. It would appear that the major predictor of health risks associated with obesity is body fat distribution. Body fat may be preferentially located in the abdomen (android pattern) or

---

[1]Sleep apnea can be central (no spontaneous respiratory effort), obstructive (respiratory effort present) or combination (mixed). Sleep apnea can be lead to severe arterial hypoxemia (decreased oxygenation of the body tissue), recurrent arousal, increased symptomatic tone, pulmonary and systemic hypertension, cardiac arrhythmias and narcolepsy. There is good evidence that symptoms of sleep apnea improve with weight loss. In addition obesity can lead to pulmonary compromise by increased weight on the thoracic case and abdomen thereby decreasing compliance of the lung.

surrounding hips and thighs (gynoid pattern). The android pattern of obesity is associated with a variety of metabolic derangements such as the metabolic syndrome. Thus, even at the same level of being overweight the individual with a greater amount of android (visceral or abdominal) fat is more likely to have or develop many of serious health conditions associated with obesity. The waist hip ratio (WHR) increases with an increase in waist circumference and is used as a measurement of abdominal adiposity. An increase in the WHR (greater than 0.8 in women and 1.0 in men) has been shown to be a better marker than BMI for the risk of death in women age 55 to 69 years.

Maternal obesity is a significant risk factor for the development of gestational diabetes mellitus and neural tube (spinal cord) defects in the fetus. Increase in body weight is associated with increased risk of cancer including colon, prostrate, endometrial and post menopausal breast cancer. An estimated 34 to 56% of endometrial cancers are attributed to a BMI of greater than 29. Almost half of the post menopausal breast cancers occur in women with a BMI greater than 29. Women gaining more than 20pounds from 18 years of age to midlife will double their risk of breast cancer compared to those whose weight remains stable.

Does weight loss resolve the diseases associated with obesity? The answer to this question is not clear. For the severely obese, gastrointestinal surgery (gastric bypass) can produce long-term weight loss. In the Swedish obese subjects (SOS) study, after 8 years the incidence of diabetes was 5 times lower in the surgical group, however, the initial improvement in hypertension dissipated to no difference as compared to those without weight loss. The primary goal of a 10% reduction in weight to be followed by at least 6 months of maintaining that loss is the stated goal of the nation's expert panel on the identification, evaluation, and treatment of the overweight or obese adult. This would equate to a 2 to 7 month increase in life expectancy, and reduce the years of life with hypertension by 1.2 to 3 years and reduce the years with type 2 diabetes by 0.5 to 1.7 years for both men and women aged 35 to 64 years with obesity. These findings have led to the expert panel to conclude: "At this time, there are no conclusive data proving that long-term intentional weight loss diminishes mortality rate or reduces the incidence of obesity-related disease in those who are moderately obese". Although studies are currently underway to assess this issue, the short-term improvements in risk factors and symptoms of disease associated with obesity would suggest a benefit for sustained weight reduction for those who are obese.

END NOTES

Introduction:

Adults prevalent to obesity are 20 and older, non-Hispanic, African American women; children are Mexican American. Hedley, Allison A., et al. (2004). Prevalence of overweight and obesity among US children, adolescents, and adults: 1999-2002. *JAMA,* 291(23), 2847-2850. National Heart, Lung and Blood Institute in cooperation with the National Institute of Diabetes and Digestive and Kidney Disease (1998). Treatment guidelines in Clinic Guidelines on the Identification, Evaluation and Treatment of Overweight and Obesity in Adults: Evidence Report. NIH publication No. 98-4098, p. 85.

Surgeon General stated obesity ranked second to cigarette smoking as the leading cause of preventable disease/death in the U.S. Health costs are about $117 billion/year. Donnelly, J.E., Hill, J.O., Jacobsen, D.J., Pottiger, Jeffrey, Sullivan, D.K., Johnson, S.L. et al. (2003) Effects of a 16-month randomized controlled exercise trial on body weight and composition in young, overweight men and women. *Arch Intern Med,* 163, 1343-1350.2/3 of those who see themselves overweight are trying to loose weight. Horm, John and Anderson, Kay. (1993). Who in America is trying to lose weight? *Ann Int. Med.,* 119(7), 672-74.

The BMI (Body Mass Index) of 18.5 to 24.9 is normal; 25 to 29.9 is overweight; 30 to 34.9 is obese; and more than, or equal to 40 is morbidly obese. NHLBI obesity education initiative expert panel on the identification, evaluation, and treatment of overweight and obesity in adults.In NIH Publication No. 98-4083, September 1998, 65.

The prevalence of obesity (BMI>30) has increased by 50% from 1991-8. Mokdad,AH,et al. (1999). The spread of the obesity epidemic in the United States, 1991-1998. *JAMA,*282(16),1519-1522.

Slightly more than 1/3 of women are trying to loose weight, 12% of men. About 1/3 of men and women are trying to maintain their weight. Serdula, M.K., Mokdad, A.H., Williamson, D.F., Galuska, D.A., Mendlein, J.M., Heath, G.W. (1999). Prevalence of attempting weight loss and strategies for controlling weight. *JAMA*, 282, 1353-1358.

The third best reported way to lose weight was to increase physical activity. Horm, John and Anderson, Kay. (1993). Who in America is trying to lose weight? *Ann Int. Med.,* 119(7), 672-74.

58% would like to loose weight only 36% follow a diet plan and 26% exercise three times per week; 60% report no regular exercise with 25% reporting no exercise at all. One-fifth think obesity is beyond their control due to genetics. Lemonick,Michael D. (2004). How we grew so big. *Time*, June 7, 2004, Time ,Inc.

Both sexes trying to loose weight the combination of eating fewer calories and exercising 150 minutes or more per week is reported to be only 1/5. Serdula, Mary K., et al. (1993). Weight control practices of US adolescents and adults. *Ann Intern Med*, 119(7pt2), 667-671. and Serdula, M.K., Mokdad, A.H., Williamson, D.F., Galuska, D.A., Mendlein, J.M., Heath, G.W. (1999). Prevalence of attempting weight loss and strategies for controlling weight. *JAMA*, 282, 1353-1358.

Footnote [2]: 44% female 15% male of high school students are trying to loose weight. 26% female and 15% male students reported trying to keep from gaining more weight. 50% of female students exercise and skip meals to control weight, while 30% of males use exercise and 18% of them skip meals to control weight. Serdula, M.K., Mokdad, A.H., Williamson, D.F., Galuska, D.A., Mendlein, J.M., Heath, G.W. (1999). Prevalence of attempting weight loss and strategies for controlling weight. *JAMA*, 282, 1353-1358.

There has been a rise in obesity depite a reduction in fat and calorie intake, with a increased sugar substitutes consumption from 1977-1988. Physically inactive individuals gain weight as compared to active ones. Weinsier, Roland L., et al. (1998). The etiology of obesity: relative contribution of metabolic factors, diet, and physical activity. *Am J Med* 105, 145-150.

Overweight/obese individuals are less likely to receive adequate health care and treated with distain and disrespect. Doctors view obese as lazy, sad, and lacking self control. Yanovski, Susan Z. (1998). Large patients and lack of preventive health care: physician or patient driven? *Arch Fam Med*, 7, 385.

The starvation of young military recruits has been extrapolated to weight loss in the obese inappropriately and has led to many misconceptions. Keys, A., et al. (1950). In *The Biology of Human Starvation*. Minneapolis: Univ. of Minnesota Press.

Average majority of participants in the National Weight Control Registry report eating a low fat, high carbohydrate, low calorie diet with high level of physical activity. The amount of exercise needed to maintain weight loss is about 2 hour a day of brink walking, 2500 to 3000 kcal per week. Wing, R.R. and Hill, J.O. (2001). Successful weight loss maintenance. *Annu Rev Nutr*, 21, 323-341.

Chapter 1:

Footnote [1]: Individuals with 100 pound weight loss where asked to chose between obesity, blindness, deaf, diabetes or amputee. No one chose to be obese again. They viewed blindness and amputation as being worse than obesity. Allison, D.B. and Saunders, S.E. (2000). Obesity in North America: an overview. *Medical Clinics of North America*, 84(2). Philadelphia: W.B. Saunders Comp. 305-332.

Television is the most widely used advertising media, adults spend 2 hours a day watching T.V. French, S.A., Story, Mary and Jeffery, R.W. (2001). Environmental influences on eating and physical activity. *Annu Rev public Health*, 22, 309-335.

Disinhitition is the loss of control following a cognitive, emotional pharmacological event. Yanovski, S.Z. and Sebring, N. G. (1994). Recorded food intake of obese women with binge eating disorder before and after weight loss. *International Journal of Easting Disorders*, 15(2), 135-150. Stunkard, A.J. and Messick, Samuel. (1985). The three-factor eating questionnaire to measure dietary restraint, disinhibition and hunger. *Journal of Psychosomatic Research*, 29(1), 71-83.

Binge eating is present in 20 to 50% of obese patients seeking treatment, where as only 2% of a community sample has this eating disorder. Yanovski, S.Z, Leet, Melissa, Yanovski, J.A., Flood, Marilyn, Gold, P.N. Kissileff, H.R., et al.(1992). Food selection and intake of obese women with binge-eating disorder. *Am J Clin Nutr*, 56, 975-980.

The incident of BED increases with the severity of obesity and is associated with early onset of obesity, frequent weight cycling (yo-yo), body shape disparagement, and psychological problems. Even among obese non-bingers with depression, those with BED have significantly more problems with mood to depression. Marcus, M.D., Wing, R.R., Ewing, Linda, Kern, Edward, Gooding, William, McDermot, Michael. (1990). Psychiatric disorders amount obese binge eaters. *International Journal of Eating disorders*, 9(1), 69-77.

Little scientific evidence for carbohydrate craving during binge eating, fats appear to be the preferential food choice. Yanovski, S.L. (1993). Binge eating disorder: Current knowledge and future directions. *Obesity Research*, 1 (4), 306-324.

Misreporting food intake and level of physical activity is more often the reason for individuals inability to lose weight. Lichtman, S.W., Pisarska, Krystyna, Berman, E.R., Pestone, Michele, Dowling, Hillary, Offenbacher, Esther, et al. (1992). Discrepancy between self-reported and actual caloric intake and exercise in obese subjects. Variability of body weight and health outcomes in the Framingham population. *N Engl J Med*, 327(27), 1893-1898.

During last 30 years reports in reduction is symptoms of depression and anxiety but no worsening in affect or mood in obese patients treated by behavior modification combined with moderate or severe caloric restriction with/without weight loss medication. National Task Force on the Prevention and treatment of Obesity (2000). Overweight, obesity and health risk. *Arch/Intern. Med,* 160, 898-904.

History of weight cycling has not been related to long term adverse psychological effects. Bartlett, S.J., Wadden, T.A. and Vogt, R.A.(1996). Psychosocial consequences of weight cycling. *Journal of Consulting and Clinical Psychology*, 64(3), 587-592.

Table I Effect of weight loss on other areas of life. Wing, R.R. and Hill, J.O. (2001). Successful weight loss maintenance. *Annu Rev Nutr*, 21, 232-341.

Problems that evolve as a result of weight loss are self, socialization and skills acquisition. Bocchieri, L.E., Mena, Maria, Fisher, B.L. (2002). Perceived psychosocial outcomes of gastric bypass surgery: A qualatative study. *Obesity Surgery*, 12,781-788.

Footnote [2] : Of the sexual abuse voiced by obese patients 13% was by incest, 9% molestation by someone outside of the family and 3% by forceful rape by a non-relative. Of these 29% had a subsequent abuse experience. 4% of obese patients "did not recall" but none of the always slender were uncertain of recall. Felitti, V.J. (1993). Childhood sexual abuse, depression and family dysfunction in adult obese patients: A case control study. *Southern Medical Journal*, 86(7), 732-736.

22% of obese patients who presented to a weight loss clinic in San Diego were conscious of using obesity to reduce sexual fears. Felitti, V.J. (1993). Childhood sexual abuse, depression and family dysfunction in adult obese patients: A case control study. *Southern Medical Journal*, 86(7), 732-736.

New social skills and skills of negotiation have to be developed for "emotional eaters". Bocchieri, L.E., Mena, Maria, Fisher, B.L. (2002). Perceived psychosocial outcomes of gastric bypass surgery: A qualatative study. *Obesity Surgery*, 12,781-788.

Weight loss is of about 35% of initial weight typically occurs following gastric bypass with a high rate of recidivism between 3 and 5 years afterwards. Brolin, Robert E. (2002). Bariatric surgery and long-term control of morbid obesity. *JAMA,*288(22),2793-6

Oprah Winfrey stated "My greatest failure was in believing that the weight issue was about weight. It's not. It's about not handling stress properly. It's about sexual abuse. It's about all the things that cause other people to become alcoholics or drug addicts". Felitti, V.J. (1993). Childhood sexual abuse, depression and family dysfunction in adult obese patients: A case control study. *Southern Medical Journal*, 86(7), 732-736.

Chapter 2:

Components of the RMR contribute at different rates in that skeletal muscle, which constitutes about 43% of the total mass in an adult, contributes only 22 to 36% of the RMR, whereas, the brain, which is only about 2% of the body mass, contributes 20 to 24% of the RMR. Other factors effect the RMR. The RMR declines with age, is higher in men and after exercise and can differ between different families as well as ethnic group. Goran, M.I. (2000). Energy metabolism and obesity. In *Medical Clinics of North America*, 84(2). Philadelphia: W.B. Saunders Company. 347-362.

Excess weight in obese people is about 75% fat and 25% FFM. Garrow, J.S (1987). Energy balance in man – an overview. *Am J Clin Nutr*, 45, 1114-1119.

Obese subjects that have lost weight have on the average a 15%to 25% decrease in energy the RMR, but a 30% decrease in 24 hour TEE as compared to others at the same weight who have not lost weight. Garrow, J.S. and Webster, J.D. (1989). Effects on Weight and Metabolic rate of obese Women on a 3.4 mj (800kcal) diet. *The Lancet*, June 24, 1429-1431.

TEF is relatively small and appears relatively constant, the major reduction in total energy requirements is attributable to the reduction in exercise related energy expenditure, and has been shown to account for 70% of the decrease in 24-hour TEE with the remaining 25-30% accounted for by the proportional decrease in FFM or RMR. Weigle, D.S., Sande, K.J., Iverius, Per-Henrick, Monsen, E.R., Brunzell, J.D. (1988).

Weight loss leads to a marked decrease in non-resting energy expenditure in ambulatory human subjects. *Metabolism*, 37(10), 930-936.

Reduced exercise-related energy expenditure (non-resting energy expenditure) of formerly obese people may be due not only to lower body weight but due to changes in the efficiency with which skeletal muscle converts chemical energy to mechanical energy. Rosenbaum,

Michael, Leibel, Rudolph, Hirsch, Jules. (1997) Obesity. *N Engl J Med*, 337(6), 396-460.

When compared to normal weight people the reduced work of movement accompanying weight loss cannot entirely explain the enhanced metabolic efficiency of reduced obese people since in most studies on the average they are still much heavier than people who have never lost weight. Yet, the per person total energy requirements are actually slightly less also. These compensatory changes can persist for four to six years after the initial weight loss, in which lower needs of energy intake are required to maintain that new weight than others at the same weight who have not lost weight. Leibiel, R.L. and Hirsch, Jules (1984). Diminished Energy requirements in reduced-obese patients. *Metabolism*, 33(2), 164-170.

The reduced individual must overcome this energy savings by an increase in exercise related activity on the order of 325-500 calories per day. This would be adding a time of walking at 3 miles per hour for 100 minutes per day if no restriction of food intake is made. Bessard, Thierry, Schultz, Yuer and Jequier, Eric. (1983) Energy Expenditure and postprandial thermogensis in obese women before and after weight loss. *American J. Clin. Nutr.*, 38, 680-693.

There is no evidence of a pre-existing metabolic or behavioral defect that results in a reduced energy expenditure state that predisposes to obesity. Prentice,A.M.,et al. (1986). High levels of energy expenditure in obese women. *British Medical J*, 292, 983-987.

Wiring jaws shut guaranteed a 26% weight loss with a 25% fall in RMR. However putting a nylon cord around the waist that could not be untied felled to prevent weight regain. Finer, Nicholas, Swan, Philip C., and Mitchell, Fred T. (1986). Metabolic rate after massive weight loss in human obesity. *Clin Sci*, 70, 396-398.

Half the decline in the 24 hour TEE could not be explained by the reduction of FFM or RMR. Ravussin,Eric, Burnand, Bernard, Schutz, Yves, and Jequier, Eric. (1985). Energy expenditure before and during energy restriction in obese patients. *Am J Clin Nutr*, 41, 753-759.

The fall in REE was larger than the loss of FFM, so the obese develop an energy savings adaption during weight loss. Valtuena, S.,et al. (1995). *Inter J of Obesity,* 19, 119-125.

Reduction of the 24 hour TEE occurs during day. deBoer, Janna O., et al. (1986). Adaptation of energy metabolism of overweight women to low-energy intake, studied with whole-body calorimeters. *Am J Clin Nutr*, 44, 585-595.and Van Dale, D., Saris, W.H.M., and Hoor, F. Ten. Weight maintenance and resting metabolic rate 18-40 months after a diet/exercise treatment. *Inter J Obesity*, 14, 347-359.

The RMR decline is not altered by exercise. Hill, James O.,et al. (1987). Effects of exercise and food restriction on body composition and metabolic rate in obese women. *Am J Clin Nutr*, 46, 622-630.

Exercise does not reverse the dietary depression of REE, which retuned to pre-exercise levels within 1 hour after exercise. Henson, Lindsey, C., Poole, David C., Donahoe, Cltde P., Heber, David. (1987). Effects of exercise training on resting energy expenditure during caloric restriction. *Am J Clin Nutr*, 46, 893-899.

RMR per unit of fat is not augmented by training. Owen, Oliver E. (1988). Resting metabolic requirements of men and women. *Mayo Clin Proc*, 63, 503-510.

RMR is independent of differences in body composition and aerobic fitness. Arciero, Paul J., Goran, Michael I., and Poehlman, Eric T. Resting metabolic rate is lower in women than in men. *J Appl Physiol*, 75,(6), 2514-2520.

RMR decline is not effected by the severity of caloric restriction. Sweeney, Mary Ellen, Hill, James O., Heller, Patricia A., Baney, Richard, and DiGirolamo, Mario. Severe vs moderate energy restriction with and without exercise in the treatment of obesity: efficieny of weight loss. *Am J Clin Nutr*, 57, 127-34.

Different components of the body contribute differently to the RMR Amajor portion of the RMR in alduts is relative constant because of the brain and liver metabolism which together consume 40% of the total. Age and regional fat distribution have no effect on RMR. Owen, Oliver E. (1988). Resting metabolic requirements of men and women. *Mayo Clin Proc*,63,503-51.

Protein turnover is not a major contributor to the disproportional decline of the RMR. vanGemert, W. G., et al. (2000). Energy, substrate and protein metabolism in morbid obesity before, during and after massive weight loss. *Internat J Obesity*, 24 711-718.

Yoyo frequency is not due to an increased efficiency in metabolism. Van Dale, Djoeke and Saris, Wim H.M.(1989). Repetitive weight loss and weight regain: effects on weight reduction, resting metabolic rate, and lipolytic activity before and after exercise and/or diet treatment. *Am J Clin Nutr*, 49, 409-416.

Self reported age of onset of obesity was not related to the change in RMR. Heshka, Stanley, Yang, Mei-Uih, Wang, Jack, Burt, Pamela, and Pi-Sunyer, F. Xavier. *Am J Clin Nutr,* 52, 981-986.

A sustained decrement in RMR accompanied weight loss and persisted despite increased calories and weight stabilization. Elliot, Diane L., Goldberg, Linn, and Bennett, William M. (1989). Sustained depression of resting metabolic rate after massive weight loss.

A reduced energy expenditure has persisted in subjects who have maintained a reduced body weight for periods ranging from 6 months to more than 4 years. Leibel, Rudolph L., Rosenbaum, Michael, and Hirsch, Jules. (1995). Changes in energy expenditure resulting from altered body weight. *N Eng J Med,* 332, 621-628.

Reduced obese have 15% lower metabolic rate than ideal weight counter part who has not loss. Amatruda, John M., Statt, Marcia C. and welle, Stephen L. (1993). Total and resting energy expenditure in obese women reduced to ideal body weight. *J Clin Invest*, 92, 1236-1242.

The implication of these findings is that a significant increase in exercise-related energy expenditure is needed to overcome this energy savings of the reduced-obese. Weigle, D.S., Sande, K.J., Iverius, Per-Henrick, Monsen, E.R., Brunzell, J.D. (1988). Weight loss leads to a marked decrease in non-resting energy expenditure in ambulatory human subjects. *Metabolism*, 37(10), 930-936.

Footnote [4]: Liebel, Rudolph l., Rosenbaum, Michael, and Hirsch, Jules. (1995). Changes in expenditure resulting from altered body weight. *N Engl J Med*, 332(10),621-628.

Gastric bypass is not associated with a drop in RMR. Flancbaum, Louis, Choban, Patricia S., Bradley,Lesley R., and Burge, Jean C. (1997). Changes in measured resting energy expenditure after Roux-en-Y gastric bypass for clinically severe obesity. *Surgery*, 122, 943-949.

There appears to be a metabolic "memory" that persists for at least six years following weight reduction against which the reduced obese individual must continue to struggle. Porier, N.B., Swanson, MS, MacDonald, K.G., Long S.B., Morris, P.G., Borwn, B.M. (1995). Who would have thought it? An operation proven to be the most effective therapy for adult-onset diabetes mellitus. *Annals of Surgery*, 222(3), 337-352.

Chapter 3

Between 1988 and 1998 health club membership grew 51% and it is interesting that this "boom" in health club membership occurred during the same time striking increases in weight gain in the population in general were observed. French, S.A., Story, Mary and Jeffery, R.W. (2001). Environmental influences on eating and physical activity. *Annu Rev public Health*, 22, 309-335.

Weight and fat loss was no different between diet alone and diet plus exercise groups. Van Dale, D., Saris, W.H.M., Schoffelen, P.F. M., and Ten Hoor, F. (1987). Does exercise give an additional effect in weight reduction regimens? *International J of Obesity*, 11, 367-375.

Adding exercise to a caloric restricted diet did not increase weight loss as fat in men or women. Hagan, RD, Upton, SJ, Wong, l., and Whitman, J. (1986). The effects of aerobic conditioning and/or caloric restriction in overweight men and women. *Med Sci Sports Exerc*,18,87-94.

Varying exercise intensity to a caloric-restricted diet did not increase fat loss. Ballor, Douglas L., McCarthy, John P., and Wilterdink, E. Joan. (1990). Exercise intensity does not affect the composition of diet- and exercise-induced body mass loss. *Am J Nutr,* 51, 142-146.

Weight loss during severe caloric restriction of a very low calorie diet of 5 weeks does not affect muscle efficiency in overweight individuals. Lemons, A.D., Kreitzman, S.N., Coxon, A. and Howard, A. (1989). Selection of appropriate exercise regimes for weight reduction during vlcd and maintenance. *International Journal of Obesity*, 13 (suppl.2), 119-123.

One can see that the exercise only increased weight; however, when exercise is added to a diet reduced by 1,000 calories per day, lean body mass (FFM) is preserved, although there was total body weight loss. Ballor, D.L., Katch, V.L, Becque, M.D., Marks, C.R. (1988). Resistance weight training during caloric restriction enhances lean body weight maintenenace. *Am J Clin Nutr*, 47, 19-25.

Preservation of FFM during weight loss with exercise is not associated with any statistically significant reduction in the decline in the RMR seen in weight loss combines results of many other studies on this topic. Ballor, D.L. and Poehlman, E.T. (1995). A meta-analysis of the effects of exercise and or dictary restriction on resting metabolic rate. *Eur J Physiol*, 71, 535-542.

Even when obese women are placed on a more severe diet of five week program of 800 kcal per day, exercise during caloric restricted weight loss did not prevent the drop in RMR and the decline in exercising subjects was not different from the decline in non-exercises. (Hill, James O.,Sparling, Phillip B., Shields, Toni W., and Heller, Patricia A. (1987). Effects of exercise and food restriction on body composition and metabolic rate in obese women. *Am J Clin Nutr*. Vol 46. 622-630.

High "substrate flux" is disrupted with dieting and therefore, the decline the in RMR associated with weight loss is not attenuated by exercise. Poehlman, E.T. (1989). A review: exercise and its influence on resting energy metabolism in man. *Medicine and Science in Sports and Exercise*, 21(5) 515-525.

Footnote [2] : Oxygen consumption is related directly to the amount of muscular work. Maximum oxygen uptake, therefore, reflexes maximum work capacity. Dale, D.C. and Federman, D.D. (2003). Diet and exeicse in *Scientific American medicine*, 1,26-38.

The diet alone group did not show such declines after exercise, therefore, burning more calories during that time than the exercise group. Krotkiewski, M., Toss, L., Bjorntory, P. and Holm, G. (1981). The effect of a very-low-calorie diet with and without chronic exercise on thyroid and sex hormones, plasma proteins, oxygen uptake, insulin and C peptide concentrations in obese women. *International Journal of Obesity*, 5, 287-293.

Oxygen uptake in the group with diet and diet plus. Krotkiewski, M., Toss, L., Bjorntory, P. and Holm, G. (1981). The effect of a very-low-calorie diet with and without chronic exercise on thyroid and sex hormones, plasma proteins, oxygen uptake, insulin and C peptide concentrations in obese women. *International Journal of Obesity*, 5, 287-293.

Exercise has no benefit on the ratio of fat loss to weight loss, although increased fat utilization occurs in very low calorie diets. Wirth, A.,Vogel, I., and Schlierf, G. (1987). Metabolic effects and body fat mass changes in obese subjects on a very-low-calorie diet with and without intensive physical training. *Ann Nutr Metab*, 31,378-386.

Chapter 4:

There is justified pessimism regarding long term weight maintenance following weight loss programs. Successful weight maintenance is defined as a weight regain of less than 6.6 pounds in two years and a sustained reduction in waist circumference of at least 1.6 inches. National Heart, Lung and Blood Institute in cooperation with the National Institute of Diabetes and Digestive and Kidney Disease (1998). Treatment guidelines in Clinic Guidelines on the Identification, Evaluation and Treatment of Overweight and Obesity in Adults: *Evidence Report. NIH* publication No. 98-4083. 85.

In an average nutritional weight loss program two years after treatment only 2% maintained the weight loss of at least 20 pounds and in an average behavioral weight loss program only 2.6% of men and 28.9% of women had maintained 100% of their weight loss after four years. Wing, R.R. and Hill, J.O. (2001). Successful weight loss maintenance. *Annu Rev Nutr*, 21, 323-341.

The exercise consisted of three times a week at about 500 calories per session for a total of 1500 calories per week. This resulted in those who were successful in maintaining a reduced body weight. Simple instruction without supervision during weight loss may not be adequate to reinforce activity changes in previously inactive subjects because only 5% of that group initiated exercise on their own. Pavlou, K.N., Krey, Suzanna and Steffee, William (1989). Exercise as an adjunct to weight loss and maintenance in moderately obese subjects. Am J Clin Nutr, 49, 1115-1123.

The addition or removal of learned exercise would appear to be a major contributing factor relative to weight maintenance. Pavlou, K.N., Krey, Suzanna and Steffee, William (1989). Exercise as an adjunct to weight loss and maintance in moderately obese subjects. *Am J Clin Nutr*, 49, 1115-1123.

Aerobic exercise does not have a stimulatory effect on metabolic rate in the post-obese or lean. Geissler, Catherine A., Miller, Derek

S. and Shah, Meena. (1987). The daily metabolic rate of the post-obese and the lean. *Am J Nutr*, 45, 914-920.

This appears to be a combination of not only a reduced metabolic rate, reduced work of movement at a lower body weight, reduced thermic effect of food also, other energy regulatory homeostatic factors not fully understood at this time. Weigle, D.S., Sande, K.J., Iverius, Per-Henrick, Monsen, E.R., Brunzell, J.D. (1988). Weight loss leads to a marked decrease in non-resting energy expenditure in ambulatory human subjects. *Metabolism*, 37(10), 930-936.; deGroot, Lisette, VanEs, A.JH. VanRaaij. J.M.A., Vogt, J.E., and Hautvast, J.G.A.J. (1990). Energy metabolism of overweight women one month and one year after an eight week slimming period. *Am J Clin Nurt*, 51, 578-583.; Sineret t al., 1985; Leibiel, R.L. and Hirsch, Jules (1984). Diminished energy requirements in reduced-obese patients. *Metabolism*, 33(2), 164-170.

Weight regain is variable and related more likely to maladaptive responses in terms of physical inactivity or excess energy intake. Weinsier, Roland L., et al. (1995). Metabolic predictors of obesity. *J Clin Invest*, 95, 980-985.

The NWCR maintenance diet resembles the moderate-fat, balanced nutrient reduction diets. Freedman, Marjorie R., King, Janet, and Kennedy, Eileen. (2001). Popular diets: a scientific review. *Obesity Research*, 9(suppl 1), 1S-40S.

The NWCR participants exercise 1 hour a day at moderate intensity. Those that regain had a decrease in exercise and a loss of disinhibition. They usually did not regain after 2-5 years. Wing, Rena R. and Hill, James O. (2001). Successful weight loss maintenance. *Annu Rev Nutr*, 21, 323-341.

Footnote [1]: In a follow up survey two years after a 500 kcal per day weight loss diet program, those who exercised (walking) more than 2000 kcal per week regained only 13% of their initial weight loss, whereas, those exercising at 1,200 kcal per week or 500 kcal per week had regained 72 and 75% of their weight loss, respectfully.

Ewbank, P.P., Darga, L.L. and Lucas, C.P. (1995). Physical activity as a predictor of weight maintenance in previously obese subjects. *Obesity Research*, 3(3), 257-263.

This intensity of exercise at a minimum ranges from as little as 60 to 75% maximum heart rate for 45 minutes per day for five days a week targeting an energy equivalent of 400 calories per session or 2000 calories per week, to as much as one to 1.3 hours a day at the same intensity level aiming for 2500 to 3000 calories per week. Schoeller, D.A., Shay, Kathjo and Kushner, R.F. (1997) How much phyiscal activity is needed to minimize weight gain in previously obese women. *Am J Clin Nutr*, 66, 551-556; Jakicic, J.M., Winters, Carena, Iang, Wei, Wing, R.R. (1999). Effects of intermittent exercise and use of home exercise equipment on adherence, weight loss and fitness in overweight women: A randomnized trail. *JAMA*, 282, 1554-1560.; Jakicic, J.M. and Gallagher, K.I. (2003). Exercise considerations for the sedentary overweight adult. *Exercise and sports sciences reviews*, 31 (2), 91-95.; Donnelly, J.E., Hill, J.O., Jacobsen, D.J., Pottiger, Jeffrey, Sullivan, D.K., Johnson, S.L. et al. (2003) Effects of a 16-month randomized controlled exercise trial on body weight and composition in young, overweight men and women. *Arch Intern Med*, 163, 1343-1350.

This intensity corresponds to the greatest fat utilization occurring at 55 to 72% of the aerobic capacity.[2] See figure 4.3. Less fat burning occurs at higher or lower rates of exercise. Achten, Juul, Gleeson, Michael and Jeukendrup, Asker (2002). Determination of the exercise intensity that elicits maximal fat oxidation. *Medicine and Science in Sports and Exercise*, 34 (1), 92-97.

A study of overweight women on reducing diets showed that short bouts of exercise vs. a single long bout a day of 40 minutes at one time resulted in a significantly greater number of exercise days and duration per week than the single long bout group. This would suggest that at short bouts of exercise may improve exercise adherence and as a result improve weight maintenance. Jakicic, J.M., Winters, Carena, Iang, Wei, Wing, R.R. (1999). Effects of intermittent exercise and use of home exercise equipment on adherence, weight loss and fitness in overweight women: A randomnized trail. *JAMA*, 282, 1554-1560.

Mean body weights in three groups of previously obese women in the year after completion of weight loss requires adding 80 minutes/day of moderate activity or 35 min./day of vigorous activity to sedentary lifestyle which far exceeds recommendations of the CDC , Am Coll of Sport Med, and the Surg Gen. Schoeller, D.A., Shay, Kathjo and Kushner, R.F. (1997) How much phyiscal activity is needed to minimize weight gain in previously obese women. *Am J Clin Nutr*, 66, 551-556.

Fat oxidation rates versus exercise intensity expressed as percentage of VO_{2max}, therefore, the greatest amount of fat burning occurs at 55% to 72% of exercise. Achten, Juul, Gleeson, Michael and Jeukendrup, Asker (2002). Determination of the exercise intensity that elicits maximal fat oxidation. *Medicine and Science in Sports and Exercise*, 34 (1), 92-97.

Chapter 5:

Sequence of metabolic events occurring with weight loss from decrease food intake occurs in a predictable and reproducible pattern. Kern, P.R., Naughton, J.L., Driscoll, C.E. and Loxtenkamp, D.A. (1982). Fasting: the history, pathophysiology and complications. *West J Med*, 137, 379-399.

A schematic of the changes in rates of glycogenolysis, gluconeogensis, lipolysis and ketogenisis that are required to maintain caloric homeostasis during the traansition from brief to prolonged fasting. Kern, P.R., Naughton, J.L., Driscoll, C.E. and Loxtenkamp, D.A. (1982). Fasting: the history, pathophysiology and complications. *West J Med*, 137, 379-399.

Footnote [6] : During a fast of more than 24 hours, muscle and fat utilization of glucose virtually creases. Kern, P.R., Naughton, J.L., Driscoll, C.E. and Loxtenkamp, D.A. (1982). Fasting: the history, pathophysiology and complications. *West J Med*, 137, 379-399.

Metabolic adaptation during the late or protein conservation phase of starvation. Saudek and Felig (1976.). The metabolic events of starvation. *The American Journal of Medicine,* Vol 60, January, 117-126.

This provides an explanation for the success of weight loss diets that include variable amounts of protein but little or no carbohydrates. Flatt, J.P. and Blackburn, G.L. (1974). The metabolic fuel regulatory system: implications for protein-sparing therapies during caloric deprivation and disease. *Am J Clin*, 27, 175-187.

Chapter 6:

However there is plenty of evidence that although lean human beings die between 57 to 73 days from starvation loosing about 40% of their body weight, there are several reports of obese individuals who have starved for more than 100 days and survived. Elia, M. (2000). Hunger disease. *Clinical Nutrition*, 19(6), 319-386.

The contribution of protein oxidation to basal metabolic rate (BMR) after various period of starvation (no energy) in lean and obese subjects. Elia, M. (2000). Hunger disease. *Clinical Nutrition*, 19(6), 319-386.

The effect of initial body mass index (left) and percent body fat on the contribution of protein oxidation to basal metabolic rate. Elia, M. (2000). Hunger disease. *Clinical Nutrition*, 19(6), 319-386.

Obese individuals will loose a much smaller proportion of lean tissue during weight loss than lean individuals on similar diets. Elia, M. (2000). Hunger disease. *Clinical Nutrition*, 19(6), 319-386.

Higher amounts of protein (80grams), however, diminish the breakdown of fat which results in a drop in ketonuria. Bolinger, R.E., Lukert, B.P., Brown, R.W., Guevara, Lila, Steinberg, Ruth, Kan, K.C. (1966). Metabolic balance of obese subjects during fasting. *Arch Intern med*, 118, 3-8.

Also shown in figure 6.6 is that dietary fat supplementation does not spare nitrogen loss but has less effect on reducing fat breakdown as carbohydrates. Bolinger, R.E., Lukert, B.P., Brown, R.W., Guevara, Lila, Steinberg, Ruth, Kan, K.C. (1966). Metabolic balance of obese subjects during fasting. *Arch Intern med*, 118, 3-8).

Plots of relative weight loss due to lean body mass in underfeeding experiments of at least 4-week duration, with subjects grouped according to midpoint body fat content and by energy intake. Prentice, A.M., Goldberg, S.J., Black, A.E., Murgatroyd, P.R. (1991). Physiological responses to slimming. *Proceedings of the Nutritional Society*, 50, 441-458.

Composition of weight loss following gastric bypass surgery. Bothie, Albert, Bistrian, B.R., Greenberg, Isaac, Blackburn, G.L. (1979). Energy regulation in morbid obesity by multidisciplinary therapy. *In Surgical Clinics of North America* (vol. 59(6). Philadelphia: W.B. Sanders Company. 1017-1030.

The effect on the nitrogen balance of starvation and of increasing amounts of protein supplementation are shown in the upper portion. Bolinger, R.E., Lukert, B.P., Brown, R.W., Guevara, Lila, Steinberg, Ruth, Kan, K.C. (1966). Metabolic balance of obese subjects during fasting. *Arch Intern med*, 118, 3-8.

These graphs show that a progressive exercise program added to a low calorie, reducing diet can result in (1) preservation of existing lean body tissue; (2) increase fat loss; (3) increase VO_2 max (or cardiovascular fitness); and (4) increase in strength, as shown with the quadriceps leg muscles. The increase strength without total body weight gain must come from recruitment of extra fibers or a redistribution of an extra protein pool. Pavlou, Konstantin N., Steffee, William P., Lerman, Robert H., and Burrows, Belton A. (1985). Effects of dieting and exercise on lean body mass, oxygen uptake, and strength. *Medicine and Science. In Sports and Exercise.* Vol 17 (4), 466-471.

One would, therefore, suspect that there are moderate lean tissue losses throughout the body and these losses are for the most part from non-muscle protein pool. Ballor, D.L., Katch, V.L, Becque, M.D., Marks, C.R. (1988). Resistance weight training during caloric restriction enhances lean body weight maintenenace. *Am J Clin Nutr*, 47, 19-25.

Ex represents the exercise group and NE represents no exercise. Konstantin Pavlou N., Steffee, William P., Lerman, Robert H., and Burrows, Belton A. (1985). Effects of dieting and exercise on lean body mass, oxygen uptake, and strength. *Medicine and Science. In Sports and Exercise.* Vol 17 (4), 466-471.

Resting metabolic rate (RMR) decreases with weight loss and is not increased with exercise training despite a substantial training induced increase in physical fitness (VO_2max) unlike what happens in those not loosing weight. (Henson, Lindsey C., Poole, David C., Donahoe, Clyde P., Heber, David. (1987). Effects of exercise training on resting energy expenditure during caloric restriction. *Am J Clin Nutr.* Vol 46, 893-909.

The total RMR decline was 19% in exercisers and 17.3% in non-exercisers at the end of the 6 week diet. Hill, James O., Sparling, Phillip B., Shields, Toni W., and Heller, Patricia A. (1987). Effects of exercise and food restriction on body composition and metabolic rate in obese women. Vol 46, 622-630.

There was improvement in the muscle endurance during the first two weeks with no further improved after another two weeks. (Krotkiewski, M., Toss, L., Bjorntory, P. and Holm, G. (1990). The effect of a very-low-calorie diet with and without chronic exercise on thyroid and sex hormones, plasma proteins, oxygen uptake, insulin and C peptide concentrations in obese women. International Journal of Obesity. Vol 5, 287-293.

Footnote[2]: Nelson, Ralph A.,et al. (1975). Nitrogen metabolism in bears: urea bladder metabolism in summer starvation and in winter sleep and role of urinary in water and nitrogen conservation. *Mayo Clin Proc*, 50,141-156.

In obese patients who have lost at least 20% of their body mass following verticalbanded gastroplasty, there was significant improvement in respiratory muscle endurance after sixmonths. Waizman, W.P., Rabner, W.M. and Zamir, M.R. (1998). Influence of excessiveweight loss after gastroplasty for morbid obesity on respiratory muscle performance. *Thorax*, 53(1), 39-42.

Chapter 7

Studies of Mexican-Americans and Pima Indians have revealed strong positional candidate genes for obesity, on chromosomes 2 and 8. Comuzzie, A.G. and Allison, D.B. (1988). The search for human obesity genes. Science, 280, 1374-1377.

Parental obesity more than doubles the risk of a child under the age of 10 years of becoming an obese adult. Among 3 to 5 year olds, the chance of adult obesity increased from 24% if neither parent was obese to 62% if at least one parent was obese. All this data on the Puget Sound study is from the same source as is Footnote 2. Whitaker, R.C., Wright, J.A., Pepe, M.S., Sedel, K.D., Dietz, W.H. (1997). Predicting obesity in young adulthood from childhood and parental obesity. N Engl J Med, 337(13), 869-873.

Although the genetic contribution was from 5 to 30% (the greater contribution for an internal fat pattern of distribution as opposed to superficial), the transmissible component from generation to generation was primarily cultural (non-genetic) and that the non-transmissible influences (environmental) usually had more important effect than the transmissible components. Bouchard, Claude, Perusse, Louis, Leblanc, Claude, Tremblay, Angeb and Theriadult, Germain. (1988). Inheritance of the amount and distribution of human body fat. International Journal of Obeisty, 12, 205-215.

In the above mentioned Danish adoptee study the estimate of heritability of BMI was 34% suggesting that the remaining variation of BMI was mostly due to non-shared environmental effects. Sorensen, T.T.A., Holst, Clause, Stunkarad, A.J., Skovgaard, L.T. (1991). Correlations of body mass index of adult adoptee and their biological and adoptive relatives. International journal of Obesity, 16, 227-236.

Footnote[3]: Neel, James V. (1962). Diabetes mellitus: a "thrifty genotype" rendered detrimental by "progress" ? Am J Hum Genet, 14, 353-362.

A schematic summary of the major affects of human variation in body composition and fat distribution. Bouchard, Claude, Perusse, Louis, Leblanc, Claude, Tremblay, Angeb and Theriadult, Germain. (1988). Inheritance of the amount and distribution of human body fat. *International Journal of Obeisty*, 12, 205-215.

With the increase in obesity, adverse health consequences emerge such as hypertension, which ranges from only about 15% in those living in Africa to over 30% among those in the United States. Jebb, S.A. (1997). Etiology of obesity. *British Medical Bulletin*, 53(2), 264-285.

Those with little physical activity however had gained weight and had twice the risk of gaining in excess of 5kg than the physically active subjects. Jebb, S.A. (1997). Etiology of obesity. *British Medical Bulletin*, 53(2), 264-285.

When controlling for food preferences, twin studies and cross cultural population studies have suggested a genetic heritability of RQ of 20 to 45%. Jebb, S.A. (1997). Etiology of obesity. *British Medical Bulletin*, 53(2), 264-285.

In experimental overfeeding of lean and obese subjects, there was no significant difference in the rate of weight gain when matched for their intake. Diaz, E., et al. (1992). *Am J Nutr*, 56, 641-655.

No evidence of a metabolic defect was found for obesity in postpartum women. Prentice, A.M., et al. (1986). High levels of energy expenditure in obese women. *British* Medical J, 292, 983-987.

Chapter 8:

There is an increase rT_3 during weight reduction secondary to decreased clearance and there is diversion of T_4 metabolism from T_3 to the less active r T_3. Kern, P.R., Naughton, J.L., Driscoll, C.E. and Loxtenkamp, D.A. (1982). Fasting: the history, pathophysiology and complications. *West J Med*, 137, 379-399.

Thyroid supplementation on very low calorie diets had the greatest tendency for curtailing weight loss and was paradoxically associated with the lowest basal metabolic rate. Moore, Ray; Howard, A.N., Grant, A.M., Mills, Ivor H. (1980). Treatment of obesity with triiodothyronine and a very-low-calorie diet liquid formula diet. *Lancet,* 223-226.

For weight loss thyroid supplementation appears to be at the expense of loss of lean tissue over fat tissue and not preferred. (Kerndt, Peter R., Naughton, James L., Driscoll, Charles E., and Loxterkamp, David A. (1982). Fasting: The history, pathophysiology and complications. *West J Med.* Vol 137, 379-399.

Despite the drop in T_3 clinical hypothyroidism does not develop during weight loss. (Glass, Allan R., (1989). Endocrine aspects of obesity. In *Med Clin Of North Am.* Vol 73 (1), Philadelphia: W.B. Saunders Comp. 139-160.

Despite the common similarities of Cushing's Syndrome to obesity there is no evidence that obesity is associated with elevated cortisol levels. Peiris, Alan and Kissebah, Ahmed (1987). Endocrine abnormalities in morbid obesity. In *Gastroenterology Clinics of North America*, Vol 16 3rd Ed. Philadelphia: W.B. Saunders Company. 389-398.

DHEA levels are normal in human obesity and administration of large doses to obese men produce no change in body weight. The topics of testosterone, growth hormone, IGF-1, footnote[2], and later CRH are derived from this source as follows. Flier, J.S. and Foster, D.W. (1998). Eating Disorders: obesity, anorexia nervosa and bulimia nervosa. *In Williams textbook of Endocrinology*, 9th Ed. Philadelphia: W.B. Saunders Company. 1061-1097.

The humoral messengers from the gut of leptin, SOCS,NYP, CCK-GIP, and GLP-1. Badman, Michael K. and Flier, Jeffery S. (2005). The gut and energy balance: visceral allies in the obesity wars. *Science*, 307, 1907-1914.

Weight loss leads to lower than expected leptin levels. Weight gain leads to expected gains in leptin levels. These findings suggest a genetic or developmental role for leptin in reproduction. Rosenbaum, Michael, Leibel, Rudolph L. and Hirsch, Jules. Obesity. *N Eng J Med*, 337(6),369-406

Ghrelin and regulation of body weight. Cummings, D.E., Weigle, D.S., Frayo, Scott, Breen, P.A., MA, M.K., Dellinger, E.P., et al. (2002) Plasma ghrelin levels after diet-induced weight loss or gastric bypass surgery. *N Engl J of Med*, 346(21), 1623-1630.

This is consistent with post gastric bypass patients reporting less feelings of hunger. Cummings, D.E., Weigle, D.S., Frayo, Scott, Breen, P.A., MA, M.K., Dellinger, E.P., et al. (2002) Plasma ghrelin levels after diet-induced weight loss or gastric bypass surgery. *N Engl J of Med*, 346(21), 1623-1630.

GIP elevations are reduced by gastric bypass.CCK response is not altered by bypass. Kellum,John M., et al. Gastroinstinal hormone responses to meals before and after gastric bypass and vertical banded gastroplasty.*Ann Surg*,211(6), 763-771.

Footnote[7]: The insulinotropic effect of GIP diminishes and the GLP-1 effect continues with the progression of diabetes. Badman, Michael K. and Flier, Jeffrey S. (2005). The gut and energy balance: visceral allies in the obesity wars. Sci, 307,1190-1914.

Rimonabant is the cannabinoid receptor antagonist. Despres, Jean-Pierre, Golay, Alain and Sjostrom, Lars (RIO- Lipid study group). (2005). Effects of rimonabant on metabolic risk factors in overweight patients with dyslipidemia. *N Engl J of Med* ,353(20), 2121-2134.

Footnote[8]: Adiponectin, cytokines, inflammatory factors, to liposuction. Also, weight increases the size and number of fat cells mentioned earlier comes from this article. Underwood, Anne and Adler, Jerry. (2004). What you don't know about fat. In *Time,* Aug. 23, 40-47: Time, Inc. Time, also, did an award winning issues on obesity in June 7, 2004, and in June 6, 2005.

This persistence of subnormal prolactin release in obese subjects which not corrected by weight loss points to the possibility of an underling hypothalamic dysfunction in obesity. Glass, Allan R. (1989) Endocrine aspects of obesity. *In Medical Clinics of North America.* Vol 73 (1). Philadelphia: W.B. Saunders Comp. 139-160.

Chapter 9:

Age adjusted death rates for ischemic heart disease declined from 345 per 100,000 in 1980 to 186.6 per 100,000 in the year 2000 Flegal, K.M., Graubard, B.I., Williamson, D.F., Gail, M.H. (2005). Excess deaths associated with underweight, overweight and obesity. *JAMA*, 293(15), 1861-1867.

Also unfit, lean men had a higher risk of cardiovascular disease (heart, stroke and/or kidney vascular disease) mortality than did obese, fit men. Lee, C.D., Blair, S.N., Jackson, A.S.1999). Cardiorespiratory fitness, body composition and all-cause and cardiovascular disease mortality in men. *A Clin Nutr*, 69, 373-380.

Therefore, an active way of life appears to have important health benefits for those who are overweight/obese. Barlow, C.E., Kohl, H.W., Gibbons, L.W., Blair, S.N. (1995). Physical fitness, mortality and obesity. *International Journal of Obesity*, 19 (suppl 4), 541-544.

Footnote [1] : Low fitness is of comparable importance to other cardiovascular disease risk factors as a strong independent predictor of mortality and cardiovascular disease death rates Wei, Ming, Kampert, J.B., Barlow, C.E., Nichaman, M.Z., Gibbons, L.W., Paffenbarger, R.S., et al.(1999). Relationship between low cardiorespiratory fitness and mortality in normal-weight, overweight and obese men. *JAMA*, 282(16), 1547-1553.

Similarly overweight, but not obese, men with one or more of the predisposed conditions have a three fold cardiovascular disease death rate and a two fold all-cause death rate than normal weight men without such conditions. Wei, Ming, Kampert, J.B., Barlow, C.E., Nichaman, M.Z., Gibbons, L.W., Paffenbarger, R.S., et al.(1999). Relationship between low cardiorespiratory fitness and mortality in normal-weight, overweight and obese men. *JAMA*, 282(16), 1547-1553.

These predisposing disease conditions are more likely with a high waist circumference (abdominal fat) and the association is greater in women than in men. Janssen, Ian, Katzmarzyk, P.T., Ross, Robert. (2002). Body mass index, waist circumference and health risk. *Arch Intern. Med.*, 162,2074-2079.

Among individuals who were moderately overweight (BMI of 26 to 29) those who lost 15% or more had more than twice the mortality risk from all-cause death than those without weight loss. Pamuk, E.R., Williamson, D.F., Serdula, M.K., Madans, Jennifer, Byers, T.E. (1993). Weight loss and subsequent death in a cohort of U.S. adults. *Ann. Intern. Med.*, 119(7pt. 2), 744-748.

However, in women with no preexisting illness, intentional weight loss is not associated with any change in mortality. Williamson, D.F.(1997). Intentional weight loss: patterns in the general population and its association with morbidity and mortality. *International Journal of Obesity*, 21(suppl 1), 514-519.

Lowest mortality rates are generally associated with mild to moderate weight gain. Andres, R.A., Muller, D.C., Sorkin, J.D. (1993). Long-term effects of change in body weight on all-cause mortality. *Ann Intern. Med.*, 119(7pt. 2), 737-743.

This was independent of their age, cholesterol, blood pressure, cigarette smoking status, alcohol intake or BMI. Lissner, Lauren, Odell, P.M., Dagostino, R.B., Stokes, Joseph, Kreger, B.E., Belanger, Albert, et al. (1991). *N Engl J Med*, 324, 1839-1844.; Ham, Peggy, Shekelle, R.B. and Stamler, Jeremiah (1989). Large fluctuations in body weight during young adulthood and twenty-five-year risk of coronary death in men. *American Journal of Epidemiology*, 129(2) 312-318.

However, what this really means is that overweight/obese individuals need to be taught skills to maintain weight loss and that prevention of relapse should become a more central focus of weight loss programs. Lissner, Lauren, Odell, P.M., Dagostino, R.B., Stokes, Joseph, Kreger, B.E., Belanger, Albert, et al. (1991). *N Engl J Med*, 324, 1839-1844.

This is consistent with studies that have shown that the probability of improved survival can be transferred from the unfit to those who become fit. Farrell, S.W., Brawn, L.A., Barlow, C.E., Cheng, Y.J., and Blair, S.N. (2002). The relation of body mass index, cardiorespiratory fitness and all-cause mortality in women. *Obesity Research*,10(6), 417-423.

Survival Probability. Barlow, C.E., Kohl, H.W., Gibbons, L.W., Blair, S.N. (1995). Physical fitness, mortality and obesity. *International Journal of Obesity*, 19 (suppl 4), 541-544.

Chapter 10

Continuum of popular diets. Riley, Rosemary E. (1999) Popular weight loss diets: health and exercise implications. In *Clinics in sports medicine.* Vol 18 (3). Philadelphia: W.B. Saunders Comp. 691-701.

Good and "bad" eicosanoids which are described as "powerful hormone like substances that control virtually all physiological functions in the body. (Riley, Rosemary E. (1999). Popular weight loss diets: health and exercise implications. In *Clinics in Sports medicine.* Vol 18 (3). Philadelphia: W.B. Saunders Comp. 691-701.

In a recent study that compared low carb, high-fat diets to low-fat, high carb diets, both types of diets reduced insulin levels in the long term, except the Atkins in which it did not significantly change. (Dansinger, M.L. et al. (2005). Comparison of the atkins, ornish, weight watchers, and zone diets for weight loss and heart disease risk reduction: a randomized trial. *JAMA.* Vol 293 (1), 43-53.

"The role of insulin in the synthesis and storage of fat has obscured its important effects in the central nervous system, where it acts to prevent weight gain, and has led to the misconception that insulin causes obesity." (Freedman, et al., (2001). Popular diets: a scientific review. *Obesity Research.* Vol 9, suppl. 1, 1s-40s. in a recent systematic review of the literature, weight loss while using low-carbohydrate diets was principally associated with decreased caloric intake and increased diet duration, but not with the reduction of carbohydrate content. Bravata, et al., (2003). Efficacy and safety of low-carbohydrate diets: A system review. *JAMA.* Vol 289 (14), 1837-1850.

One would suspect then that there would be variable weight loss in that the lowest carbohydrate diet would loose more than the high content diet. However, weight loss was the same for all. Golay, Alain et al. (1996). Weight-loss with low or high carbohydrate diet? *International Journal of Obesity.* Vol 20, 1067-1072. and Golay,

Alain (1996) Similar weight loss with low-or high-carbohydrate diets. *Am. J. Clin. Nutr.* Vol 63, 174-178.

For each diet, decreased cardiac risk factors of lower total/HDL cholesterol, C-reactive protein (an inflammation marker), and insulin were significantly associated with the weight loss but no significant difference with which diet was consumed. Dansinger, M.L. et al. (2005). Comparison of the atkins, ornish, weight watchers and zone diets for weight loss and heart disease risk reduction: a randomized trial. *JAMA.* Vol 293 (1), 43-53.

The low carbohydrate diets were unrestricted to the amount of calories eaten, while in most studies the high carbohydrate (low fat) dieters were also instructed on caloric restriction. Yet weight loss was usually the same. Brehm, Bonnie J., Seeley, R.J., Daniels, S.R. and D'Alessio, D.A. (2003) A randomized trial companying a very low carbohydrate diet and calorie-restricted low fat diet on body weight and cardiovascular risk factors in healthy women. *J Clin Endocrinol Medtab.* Vol 88, 1617-1623; Stern, et al,. 2004.; Yancy et al., 2004)

Diets recommended by various national health organizations for chronic disease prevention are low in fat and high in carbohydrate. Howard, B.V. et al. (2006). Low-fat dietary pattern and weight change over 7 years: the women's health initiative dietary modification trial. *JAMA.* Vol 295 (1), 31-49.

Harvard School of Public Heath which had originally suggested that fat intake may play a role in obesity, has now proposed that reducing the percent of energy intake from fat will have no important benefits on obesity and could further exacerbate the problem. Furthermore, the emphasis on fat reduction has been a serious distraction in efforts to control obesity. Acheson, K.J. (2004). Carbohydrate and weight control: where do we stand? *Curr Opin Clin Nutr Metab Care*, 7, 485-492.

Compared with low-GI meals, high GI meals induce a greater rise and fall in blood glucose and with the resultant greater rise in blood insulin there is a lowering of the   concentrations of the body's two main fuels (blood glucose and fatty acids) in the immediate post-digestive period. It is proposed that the reduced availability of metabolic fuels may act as a signal to stimulate more eating. Foster-Powell, Kaye, Holt, S.H.A. and Brand-Miller, J.C. (2002). International table of glycemic index and glycemic load values: 2002. *Am J Clin Nutr*, 76, 5-56.

It appears that the low-GI cereal had 3.5 times more protein, which probably explained the rapid insulin response and attenuated glycemic response. Acheson, Kevin J. (2004). Carbohydrate and weight control: where do we stand? *Curr Opin Clin Nutr Metab Care*, 7, 485-492.

However, obese subjects fail to sense the drop in energy density[2] and continue to consume the same volume or weight of food with resultant weight loss due to the fewer calories consumed. Campbell, et al., (1971). Studies of food-intake regulation in man: responses to variations in nutritive density in lean and obese subjects. *NEJM*, 285, 1402-07.

The major determents of dietary energy density (ED) are water and fat with ED falling as water content rises and as fat content falls. Protein and carbohydrates contribute relatively little to ED. Stubbs, James, Ferres, Steve and Horgan, Grahm (2000). Energy density of foods: effects on energy intake. *Crit Rev in Food Sci and Nutr*, 40, 481-515.

In one study men were given different volumes of equal energy content and macronutrients before lunch. Those who consumed the larger volume ate less not only for lunch, but also at the following evening meal. Rolls, et al, (1998). Volume of food consumed affects satiety in men. *Am J Clin Nutr*, 67, 1170-77.

When water is incorporated into a food (such as adding water to a casserole to make a soup) the energy intake (calories) at the meal is reduced and is not subsequently increased as the next meal. Rolls, B.J., Bell, E.A., and Thorwart, M.L. (1999). Watet incorporated into a flood but not served with a food decreases energy intake in lean women. *Am J Clin Nutr*, 70, 448-55.

When there is no restriction on the amount of food eaten, the consumption of an additional 14 grams/day of fiber for more than 2 days is associated with a 10% decrease in energy intake (calories) and body weight loss of 4 pounds over 3.8 months. Howarth, N.C., Saltzman, Edward, and Roberts, S.B. (2001). Dietary fiber and weight regulation. *Nutr Rev*, 59, 129-139.

Footnote [3]: A very conservative estimate of 2860 calories/day for an individual younger than 50 years who weighs 220lbs with a sedentary lifestyle. Eckel, R.H. (2005) The dietary approach to obesity: is it the diet or the disorder? *JAMA*. Vol 293 (1), 96-97.

Dietary intakes of National Weight Control Registry enrollees by method of weight loss. Table 10.2 Characterization of diets used for weight loss and weight maintenance. Both tables from Freedman, et al., (2001). Popular diets: a scientific review. *Obesity Research*. Vol 9 (suppl. 1), 1s-40s.

The high vitamin and calcium intake of the successful weight loss maintenance diet suggests that they eat a diet high in fruits, vegetables and dairy products. The low iron intake suggests low intake of red meats. Freedman, et al.(2001). Popular diets: a scientific review. *Obesity Research*, 9 (suppl 1), 1S-40S.

Obesity results from a disregulation of appetite and energy metabolism, which is influenced by genetics, physiologic, biochemistry, environmental and psychosocial factors. Achieving and maintaining a healthy weight are the most important criteria of any plan." Riley, Rosemary E. (1999). Popular weight loss diets: health and exercise implications. In *Clinics in Sports Medicine*, vol 18(3), Philadelphia: W.B. Saunders Comp., 691-701.

Less than half of doctors in 2006 believe that obesity is a disease. Yet, 95% know, but do not prescribe weight loss medication. Forman-Hoffman, Valerie, Little, Amanda, and Wahls, Terry. (2006). Barriers to obesity management: a pilot study of primary care clinicians. *BMC Family Practice*, http://www.biomedcentral.com/1471-2296/7/35.

Chapter 11

An Inconvenient Truth is copyrighted by Paramount Classics, a division of Paramount Pictures, 2006.

Appendix I

In a study of obese individuals applying for a weight loss program, almost half had major depression or an anxiety disorder. Marcus, M.D., Wing, R.R., Ewing, Linda, Kern, Edward, Gooding, William, McDermot, Michael. (1990). Psychiatric disorders amount obese binge eaters. *International Journal of Eating disorders*, 9(1), 69-77.

The dogs could not be coxed away from the shock; only forcibly dragging the dog to safety could the painful shocks be terminated. McKinney, W.T. (2003). Animal research and its relevance to psychiatry. *In Kaplan and Sadock's Comprehensive Textbook of Psychiatry* Vol. 1. Philadelphia: Lippincott Williams and Wilkins. pp. 545-552.

Experiences of loss and abandonment produce a dependent type of depression, whereas, experience of invalidation produce a self-critical depression. Wolfe, Barry E. (2005). Perspectives on anxiety disorders. In *Understanding and Treating Anxiety Disorders*. Washington DC: American Psychological Association. , 25-39.

Experiences of loss and abandonment produce a dependent type of depression, whereas, experience of invalidation produce a self-critical depression. Wolfe, Barry E. (2005). Perspectives on anxiety disorders. In *Understanding and*

Treating Anxiety Disorders. Washington DC: American Psychological Association,. 25-39.

The anxiety state is associated with helplessness that results in one's inability to predict or control outcomes, characterized prominently by negative evaluation of one's ability to cope. Wolfe, Barry E. (2005). Perspectives on anxiety disorders. In *Understanding and Treating Anxiety Disorders*. Washington DC: American Psychological Association, 25-39.

Appendix II

The primary conclusion from her research was that solid foods could be eaten by infants and young children and their appetite was a reliable guide for the amount of food, "not the nutritional quality". This was also confirmed by a resent study in 1991. Birch, L.L., Johnson, S.L., Anderson, Graciela, Peters, J.C., Schulte, M.C. (1991). The Variability of young children's energy intake. *N Engl J Med*, 324(4), 232-235.

Deciding how much food to consume should be the purgative of the child. However, the selection of the diet should be balanced and nutritious made by the parents and not offered to reward or punish certain kinds of behavior. Story, Mary and Brown, J.E. (1987). Sounding board: Do young children instinctively know what to eat? The studies of Clara David revisited. *N Engl J med*, 316(2), 103-105.

Appendix III

The glycogen from the muscle and liver is in short supply, too and would provide enough energy to sustain running for only six miles, while fat (adipose tissue) could possibly provide enough energy to run from Boston to Atlanta for an average weight person. Dale, D.C. and Federman, D.D. (2003). Diet and exeicse. In *Scientific American medicine*, 1,26-38.

As a result blood glucose can supply as much as 30% of the metabolic needs of exercising muscle thus sparing muscular glycogen to some extent. Dale, D.C. and Federman, D.D. (2003). Diet and exeicse. In *Scientific American medicine*, 1,26-38.

There is a capacity to increase free fatty acid utilization with prolonged exercise. This is accomplished by endurance training through increased activity of LPL in adipose and muscle tissues. Nikkila, E.A., Taskinen, M.R., Seppo, Rehunen, Harkonen, Matti. (1979) Lipoprotein lipase activity in adipose tissue and skeletal muscle of runners: relation to serum lipoproteins. *Metabolism*, 27(11), 1161-1671.

Muscle glycogen content can be dependent on the type of diet before exercise. Bergstrom,J., Hermansen,L., Hultman,E. and Saltin,B.(1967). Diet, muscle glycogen and physical performance. *Acta Physiol Scand*, 71, 140-150

Enhanced glycogen synthesis with high carb diet following exercise depletion. Mole, Paul A. (1990). Impact of energy intake and exercise on resting metabolic rate. *Sports Medicine*, 10(2), 72-87.

The use of caffeine as a potential ergogenic aid. Hawley, John A. (1998). Fat burning during exercise: can ergogenics change the balance? *The Physician and Sportsmedicine*,26(9), 56-63.

Hydroxycitric acid does not induce weigth loss. Heber, David (2003). Herbal preparations for obesity: are they useful? *Prim Care Clin Office Pract*,30, 441-463.

There is a lack of sustained elevation of RMR with training exercises. Intensity of exercise elevates RMR for short periods of time. Mole, paul A. (1990). Impact of energy intake and exercise on resting metabolic rate. *Sports Medicine*, 10(2), 72-87.

High or low exercise intensity produced the same amount of fat loss (80%) in the obese.(This loss was due to the diet.) Ballor, Douglas L., McCarthy, John P., and Wilterdink, Joan E. (1990). Exercise intensity does not affect the composition of diet- and exercise-induced body mass loss.*Am J Clin Nutr*,50, 142- 146.

Footnote[4]: Poehland, Eric T. (1989). A review: exercise and its influence on resting energy metabolism in man. *Med and Sci in Sports and Exerc*, 21(5), 515-525.

There is a paradoxical drop in metabolic rate with exercise during weight loss. Also seen in soldiers. Phinney,Stephen D., LaGrange, Betty M., O'Connell, Maureen, and Danforth,Jr, Elliot. (1988). Effects of aerobic exercise on energy expenditure and nitrogen balance during very low calorie dieting. *Metabolism*, 37(8), 758-765.

Appendix IV

In 1991 the estimated number of annual deaths due to obesity among U.S. adults was about 280,000. Allison, D.B., Fontaine, K.R., Manson, J.E., Stevens, June, Vanitallie, T.B. (1999). Annual deaths attributable to obesity in the United States. *JAMA*, 282(16), 1530-1538.

Footnote [1] : Sleep apnea can be central, obstructive or combination. Sleep apnea can be lead to severe atrial hypoxia, recurrent arousal, increased symptomatic tone, pulmonary and systemic hypertension, cardiac arrhythmias and narcolepsy. National Task Force on the Prevention and treatment of Obesity (2000). Overweight, obesity and health risk *Arch/Intern. Med,* 160, 898-904.

Most of the increase in mortality is due to cardiovascular causes, such as, heart attack, hypertension or renal vascular disease. National Task Force on the Prevention and treatment of Obesity (2000). Overweight, obesity and health risk *Arch/Intern. Med,* 160, 898-904

Thus, even at the same level of being overweight the individual with a greater amount of android (visceral or abdominal) fat is more likely to have or develop many of serious health conditions associated with obesity. National Task Force on the Prevention and treatment of Obesity (2000). Overweight, obesity and health risk *Arch/Intern. Med,* 160, 898-904.; Janssen, Ian, Katzmarzyk, P.T., Ross, Robert. (2002). Body mass index, waist circumference and health risk. *Arch Intern. Med.*, 162,2074-2079.

An increase in the WHR (greater than 0.8 in women and 1.0 in men) has been shown to be a better marker than BMI for the risk of death in women age 55 to 69 years. Solomon, Caren G. and Manson, JoAnn E. (1997). Obesity and mortality: a review of the epidemic data. *Am J Clin Nutr*, 66(suppl), 1044S-1050S.

Women gaining more than 20 pounds from 18 years of age to midlife will double risk of breast cancer compared to those whose weight remains stable. Janssen, Ian, Katzmarzyk, P.T., Ross, Robert. (2002). Body mass index, waist circumference and health risk. *Arch Intern. Med.*, 162,2074-2079.

In the Swedish obese subjects (SOS) study, after 8 years the incidence of diabetes was 5 times lower in the surgical group, however, the initial improvement in hypertension dissipated to no difference as compared to those without weight loss. Torgerson, J.S. and Sjostrom, L.(2001). The swedish obese subjects (sos) study- rationale and results. *International J of Obesity*,25 (suppl 1), s2-s4.

The reductions in life expectancy, hypertension, and diabetes with a 10% weight loss. Oster, Gerry et al. (1999). Lifetime health and economic benefits of weight loss among obese persons. *Am J Public Health*, 89, 1536-1542. This reference was choosen over the recent studies of Fontaine et al. (*JAMA*,2003,289,187-193.) and Peeters et al. (*Ann Intern Med*, 2003,138,24-32) which both have problems with their analysis of cohorts.

"At this time, there are no conclusive data proving that long-term intentional weight loss diminishes mortality rate or reduces the incidence of obesity-related disease in those who are moderately obese". National Task Force on the Prevention and treatment of Obesity (2000). Overweight, obesity and health risk. *Arch/Intern. Med,* 160, 898-904.

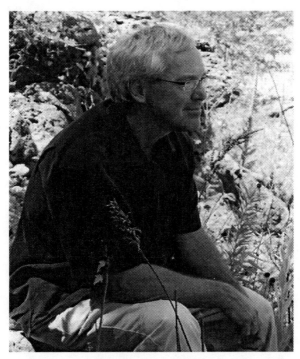

Dr. Snead has been Board Certified in Internal Medicine, Geriatrics and Bariatric Medicine. He has been practicing for more than two decades and continues to reach for excellence. He has dedicated himself for the past decade on the obesity dilemma that has gripped western societies. There is a saying that one can recognize a pioneer in his field by the number of arrows in his back. Al Gore, former vice-president of the USA, has said, "I have seen scientists who were persecuted, ridiculed, and deprived of jobs/income simply because the facts they discovered led to an inconvenient truth that they insisted on telling." Despite the arrows of arrogance and ignorance, Dr. Snead has persisted in exposing many of the myths of weight loss that have mislead so many, not only in society but many in the field of medicine. Old myths die hard and many presented here have come directly from patients that have been helped by Dr. Snead. The many years of experience and great depth of knowledge have provided Dr. Snead exceptional insight into the obesity epidemic that has come to plague so many.

Printed in the United States
118179LV00003B/502-609/A

9 781434 315984